Coping with Prolonged Health Impairment
in Your Child

Audrey T. McCollum, M.S.

Research Associate in Social Work
Department of Pediatrics
Yale University School of Medicine

Coping with Prolonged Health

Impairment in Your Child

Little, Brown and Company, Boston

Preface

It is estimated that at least 10 percent of children in the United States are afflicted with physical disorders lasting three months or longer. Many of the disorders are serious; some are dangerous. Parents of an ill or disabled child may find themselves treading a tightrope between hope and despair, perhaps for many years. Their standard and style of living may be affected significantly; every relationship within the family may be influenced.

A child whose health is impaired is nonetheless a maturing, changing child. Whether his disorder is of long standing or newly acquired, it will have special emotional, intellectual, and social meaning for the child and his family in each successive stage of his development. New issues, new reactions, and new challenges will continue to arise. And these challenges are remarkably similar whether the child's disorder affects his heart, lungs, kidneys, pancreas, blood, bones, muscles, or other bodily structures and functions.

The quality of life is as meaningful as its duration, or more so. Although parents have limited influence over the length of their child's life, there is much they can do to enhance its quality. There is much they can do to help their child believe that he is a valued human being, different from certain others because of his affliction but no less worthwhile. There is much they can do to help their child form satisfying relationships and develop his capabilities as fully as possible. Even one whose life span must be relatively brief can leave as significant an imprint on human history as one who lives to a venerable and perhaps bleak old age.

This book has been prepared to help families accomplish these awesome tasks. It cannot be absorbed in a swift, cover-to-cover reading. Rather, it is a book for reference, a book to explore and reflect on when particular behavioral, emotional, or social issues arise. It is a book to guide parents in anticipating needs and planning solutions. It is a book that makes available to families the composite experience of countless others who have faced similar problems and found effective ways of coping. It describes the often unrecognized ways in which professional persons—clergymen, dietitians, educators, inhalation therapists, nurses, occupational therapists, physicians, physiotherapists, psychologists, social workers, vocational counselors—can offer significant help to child and family.

This is, in part, a painful book. It is, however, based on the conviction that profound challenge—and the threatened loss of a child is surely among the most profound—can arouse the latent strength in human character. Most parents can master this challenge. Most parents do.

A. McC.

New Haven, Connecticut

Acknowledgments

This book has been based in part on experience with patients and their families in the Yale Children's Clinical Research Center (supported by grant RR-00125, General Clinical Research Centers Program, National Institutes of Health) and the Yale Cystic Fibrosis Program (supported by grants from the National Cystic Fibrosis Research Foundation and the Department of Health, of the state of Connecticut). In addition, the author benefited greatly from the observations of other professional workers concerned with the social and emotional aspects of chronic or life-threatening medical disorders of childhood. These observations were found in a survey of the professional literature published between 1948 and 1973.

The author is deeply appreciative of the helpful comments and suggestions made by colleagues in nursing, pediatrics, psychiatry, and social work who reviewed sections of the manuscript. These include: Ruth L. Breslin, M.S.W., Marie Browne, M.D., Charles D. Cook, M.D., Sheila G. Cook, M.S., Kathryn M. Dyer, M.S.W., Myron Genel, M.D., Paul S. Goldstein, M.D., Y. Edward Hsia, M.D., Leonard S. Krassner, M.D., Melvin Lewis, M.D., Ruth D. Lord, M.A., Roberta S. O'Grady, R.N., M.A., Ellis A. Perlswig, M.D., Sally A. Provence, M.D., Julina P. Rhymes, R.N., M.S.N., Joseph D. Saccio, M.D., A. Herbert Schwartz, M.D., Ruth L. Silverberg, M.S.W., Albert J. Solnit, M.D., and Morris A. Wessel, M.D.

A uniquely valuable contribution was made by several parents of children with impaired health who reviewed the manuscript from the perspective of their personal experiences. These parents are: Mr. and Mrs. John Birkenberger, Mrs. Robert N. Margolis, Mrs. Brian Molloy, and Mr. and Mrs. Robert Washburn.

In addition, the author is extremely grateful to the following for their kindness in reviewing the manuscript: Bruce D. Bennett, Special Consultant for the Respiratory Disease Program, American Lung Association; Mrs. R. Samuel Howe, Vice-President, American Lung Association; Gregory Kaye, Executive Director, Cystic Fibrosis Association of Connecticut; Philip Nelbach, Executive Director, Connecticut Diabetes Association; Paul R. Patterson, M.D., Director, Pediatric

Pulmonary Disease Center, Albany Medical College; and Harlan Stricklett, Planning Associate, American Lung Association.

Throughout the preparation of the manuscript, dedicated and skillful secretarial assistance was provided by Patricia Wislocki.

Contents

Preface   *v*
Acknowledgments   *vii*

1   Facing the Diagnosis   **1**
     First Responses   *1*
     Grief   *3*
     Guilt   *4*
     Anger   *9*
     Apprehension and Anxiety   *13*

2   Safeguarding Family Relationships   **21**
     Your Marriage   *21*
     Your Other Children   *25*
     Grandparents   *32*

3   Coping with Impaired Health in the Infant and Toddler   **37**
     Baby's Needs and Your Grief   *37*
     The Feeding Experience   *39*
     Bodily Movement and Activity   *42*
     Assertiveness and Home Treatment   *47*
     Impulse Control   *50*
     Hospitalization and the Separation Experience   *53*

4   Coping with Impaired Health in Early Childhood   **59**
     Family Relations: Tenderness and Rivalry   *59*
     Fact and Fancy   *64*
     Communication through Language   *72*
     Play   *75*
     Widening Social Horizons   *78*
     Hospitalization   *82*

5   Coping with Impaired Health in Mid-Childhood   **93**
     Being Different   *93*
     The Sense of Accomplishment   *101*
     Explaining the Illness   *110*
     Managing the Medical Regimen   *120*
     Hospitalization   *127*

6   Coping with Impaired Health in Adolescence   **135**

The Challenges   136
Helping the Teenager Cope   144
Hospitalization   161
The "Battered" Parent   169

7   Should You Have Another Baby?   **173**

Risks to the Parent-Child Relationship   173
Risk of Recurrence   175
Preventing Pregnancy   175
Interrupting Pregnancy   178
Predicting the Outcome   180
Alternate Routes to Parenthood   182

8   Sources of Help   **185**

Effective Teamwork with the Doctor   185
Crucial Questions   191
Inherited Illness and Genetic Counseling   205
Personal Counseling and Psychotherapy   211
Parent Groups   213
Voluntary Health Agencies   218
Social Action   222
Financial Resources   226
Satisfactions Outside Parenthood   228

Appendix: Service Organizations   231
Index   235

To Bob, Cindy, and Doug
Each of whom contributed in a very special way to this work

1

Facing the Diagnosis

How do parents feel when faced with the threat of serious illness or disability in their child? Is it helpful to know what others have experienced? Many parents believe it is. Knowing how others have felt in similar circumstances can reduce the sense of being utterly alone. It can help parents recognize that their own feelings and reactions are appropriate, and reduce their concern about being different, unnatural, or even "crazy." It can help parents communicate their emotions and needs to others. It can help relatives and friends find ways to be genuinely supportive and helpful.

First Responses

Everyone must find his own pace in coming to terms with a painful truth. So it is for you as the parent of a child whose health is impaired. You may need to thrust that truth away — to ward it off — until, little by little, you can bear to take it in. When the doctor confronts you with the awful fact of your child's illness (as gentle as the doctor may be, it is still an awful confrontation), you may not believe him. You may be certain that he's quite mistaken about your child — it couldn't possibly be what he says it is. Or else, the whole scene may seem unreal; you can't believe it's really happening to you.

You may not be able to grasp what he's telling you. It's as though your mind is a TV screen that keeps going blank. You hear the words and then they're gone. After the conference, it may be almost impossible to remember what the doctor did say, or you may be convinced that he didn't really explain anything much at all.

You may feel nothing at all. As you listen to the doctor's words, they may seem real, they may make sense, you may believe him and even ask questions — but in a strange, detached way as though you're talking not about your own child but about some textbook case. It may seem not to affect you much.

Refusing to believe the diagnosis, putting it out of your mind by forgetting, or thinking and talking about it without emotion are common responses that can either help or hinder you in coming to terms with your child's condition. It is natural to wish desperately to fight a worrying diagnosis, to prove the doctor wrong and be able to find a different answer. Why should a parent accept disturbing news meekly? However, a sense of trust in the doctor will be one of the most important elements in helping you meet the challenge of your child's illness, and for this reason it is essential to resolve the first doubts. A wise doctor is prepared for the fact that many parents do experience a period of disbelief. Should your disbelief lead you to refuse treatment for your child (parents rarely do), the doctor will be disturbed and concerned for your child's safety. However, if you share your doubts with him, it is likely that he will understand and sympathize, and may suggest a consultation with another physician or in another medical center. Should he fail to suggest a consultation, it is appropriate for you to request one if it would help you and if it could be carried out without hardship to your child.

Forgetting is a common and understandable defense against emotional pain. Bright people, average people, and slow people all deal with anguish by forgetting. Parents, however, often view forgetting what the doctor has said as a sign of their own inadequacy, and feel shy and apologetic about asking the doctor to repeat what he has explained before. Such a request is difficult the first time one forgets, but almost impossible the second, third, or fourth time. It may seem easier to ask questions of friends, relatives, or even the neighborhood pharmacist, none of whom are likely to be fully qualified to give accurate, complete medical information. Or a parent may go to the nearest library and try to read up on the disease in a reference book that may be years out of date and offers no information about recent advances in the treatment of the illness.

Mrs. A.'s nine-year-old daughter was examined in a medical center because of a cough that had persisted for several years. A specialist had discussed with Mrs. A. the possibility that her daughter had a chronic lung condition, cystic fibrosis, and had explained the nature of the disease. A special test was performed, and since the result would not be available for several days, it was arranged that Mrs. A. would be notified by telephone. The test did confirm the diagnosis, and Mrs. A. was called and informed. She was stunned and unable to ask questions. After she had hung up, she realized that she could remember nothing of what the doctor had told her earlier about the disease except its name. She had forgotten his reassurance that the condition was not far advanced in her daughter and that the outlook for keeping it under control was quite hopeful. Alone at home and panic stricken, she could make no decision about where to turn for information or comfort. Finally, she walked to a nearby drugstore for aspirin and asked the druggist if he had heard of cystic fibrosis. "It's funny you should ask," he said, "because there's a lady right over there who knows a lot about it." Mrs. D., that lady, did indeed know, but her knowledge was derived from a tragic loss. When the illness was identified in her own child, it had been far too advanced for treatment to be effective. Mrs. A.'s shy questions loosed a deluge of Mrs. D.'s anguish and bitterness. Mrs. A. was overwhelmed by a terrifying — and incorrect — belief that this was what lay in store for her also. No amount of later reassurance could eradicate the fear left from this searing encounter.

In such a fashion, parents may expose themselves to information that is incorrect, out of date, and much more frightening than what the doctor would have given. It is legitimate and important to let the doctor know that your anxiety made it hard to remember what he told you, and to ask him for further conferences. If this is difficult for him to arrange, it is reasonable to ask him to designate another professional person toward whom you can direct your questions. You will need, and you deserve, such opportunities again and again.

Parents whose feelings become sealed off in response to acute stress are sometimes mistakenly judged to be cold and uncaring. Such a parent may appear so competent that his inner needs can readily be overlooked. His detachment, lack of emotional display, and perhaps even a rather intellectual approach to the child's problem may encourage physicians to communicate with him as though he were a professional colleague rather than a parent (perhaps explaining too much too quickly and in overly technical language). If you, or your spouse, are such a person, it may be difficult indeed to let others know the extent of your hidden anguish. However, others may at least need to be reminded that although your grief is not obvious, you are not uncaring about your child. It will also be essential for you to allow yourself opportunities for the gradual release of your feelings.

Whatever first responses have shielded you a little from anguish about your child's disorder, sooner or later — slowly or in a deluge — your feelings will make themselves known. What are you likely to feel when faced with the threat of serious health impairment in your child?

Grief

Grief is concerned with loss — loss that has already occurred, loss that is imminently expected and loss that is feared in the future. When a child develops a threatening illness, grief is inevitable for those who care about him. A parent grieves not only for the feared loss of the child but also for the loss of certain hopes and dreams for him. One cannot have quite the same expectations for a child with kidney or heart or lung disease, a child with anemia or diabetes or epilepsy or cancer, that one has for a healthy child. Some hopes will need to be modified, some must be given up altogether. And so there is grief in the beginning of the illness and grief again at later times when the parents are faced with changing aspects of the child's condition.

Grief is an intermingling of feelings that can rage fiercely. Grief is wild despair. Grief is bitter remorse. Grief is burning anger, clutching fear. Grief is sorrow, a leaden sadness of such a weight that your body feels weary and moves slowly and with great effort. The world around you may seem gray, drab, uninteresting. It doesn't matter what the weather is like, whether you bother to comb your hair, what you eat for lunch or whether you eat lunch at all. Your eyes sting and your throat aches with unshed tears. Grief is exhausting and disorganizing. You may find yourself forgetting things and doing things that don't quite make sense. Simple decisions may be hard to reach, and you may be unable to keep your mind on the task at hand. You may feel intensely irritable, ready to fly apart into a thousand pieces.

There are places in the world where grief is openly shared. It is released in keening, wailing, weeping, in songs of lamentation and in dance. Our society of youth, vigor and smiling faces insists that grief should be a private matter. Women may weep, but have them weep quietly and in solitude. Men? Be brave, they are urged; their grief should be concealed altogether. And so, grief is isolating.

But grief is concerned with loss, and for this very reason human closeness, a sense of relatedness to others, is needed for comfort. The bonds that develop between those who grieve together may, in fact, have a special depth. Just to be with a person who cares, who may convey his concern through nothing more than a glance or a touch of the hand, offers solace. However, to relieve the intensity of grief there must also be release in words and in tears.

There is no length of time one should grieve. This depends on many things, including the nature of your child's disorder, your special feelings about him, other relationships in your family, and your own personality. There is no special way one should feel. There is, however, a range of feelings a grieving parent is likely to experience, and a variety of ways in which a parent may cope with these feelings.

Guilt

There are few human emotions as tormenting as guilt, yet most parents of sick children seem destined to experience guilt to some degree. In fact, some parents virtually place themselves on trial, playing the roles of accused, prosecuting attorney, judge, and jury. An attorney for the defense may never be appointed at all (would you tolerate such treatment if you were summoned to court for a traffic offense?). The nature of the verdict, that is, whether self-accusation finally gives way to self-forgiveness, will be one of the most crucial elements in your adjustment to your child's illness. A chronically guilt-laden parent is a parent unable to like or respect himself. He will have difficulty helping his child maintain his own feelings of worth and dignity. He may seek ways to atone for his guilt, perhaps through lavishing excessive attention and care on the child (who is almost certain, then, to become unhappily aware that he is a burden). The parent will scarcely be able to help other members of the family master the enormous challenge of the illness. What, then, are some of the guilt-laden ideas that parents have — that perhaps you have?

Feeling Responsible for the Illness

Parents expect themselves to keep their children safe. When children are found to be ill, the same uneasy questions come to the mind of almost every parent: "Is it my fault? Could I have prevented it if I'd cared for my child in a different way or a better way, or if I'd been a better person?"

Jerry was a jaunty nine-year-old who much preferred fishing to phonetics. Although he had the sniffles, he persuaded his mother one bright September afternoon to let him go to the lake to try out a new rod. Lucky in his catch, Jerry was heedless running home. He stumbled on one of the stepping stones that crossed the stream feeding the lake, toppled in, and was soaked. Three days later, Jerry was desperately ill with high fever and coma. The diagnosis: inflammation of the brain probably caused by a virus. In an agony of fear that Jerry would never fish again, his mother reproached herself over and over: "The soaking on top of his sniffles must have brought on the fever. If only I hadn't let him go."

Priscilla's parents were harassed. Chronically worried about providing for five children, chronically weary from long days of work, they felt increasingly irritable and dissatisfied with each other. Their arguments became more frequent, noisier, more bitter. When Priscilla was four, she developed leukemia. It was many weeks before her mother, desperately dreading but also needing the answer, could put into words this question: "Some time ago I heard or read somewhere — I can't remember which — that leukemia can be brought on by emotional upsets. Priscilla has always been high strung and sensitive. Could she have gotten sick because Ed and I were fighting so much?"

Dave and Dorothy were teenagers whose parents strongly opposed their wish to marry. Believing that they could force their parents to give consent if Dorothy became pregnant, the young couple had frequent sexual relations, and Dorothy did become pregnant. The marriage took place (with their parents' angry and grudging consent). The baby, born seven months later, had a seriously defective heart. Dorothy was grieved, but Dave was devastated. Already troubled because his premarital sexual activity had violated the strict moral standards of his family and the teachings of his Church, he became convinced that his baby's illness had been inflicted by God as punishment for his sin. His guilty anguish was intensified because it was the baby, not he, who suffered physically.

In none of these cases were the parents at all responsible for their children's illnesses. In time, they came to accept that, helped by explanations and reassurance from the doctors.

Some disorders are inherited, passed from one generation to the next in a pattern determined by certain biological laws.* Sometimes no family history has been recognized before. Parents may be quite unaware of carrying a particular genetic trait until a disorder is identified in one of their offspring. None are morally or psychologically responsible for the biological inheritance that they receive and, in turn, pass on. But it is hard for these parents to avoid at least a temporary feeling of having done something bad to the afflicted child. Sometimes the thought is of this nature: "I'm an inadequate person because I do have this trait in my genetic makeup, and my inadequacy has caused my child this illness."

On occasion parents do know of the existence of the genetic trait, but decide to take a chance on bearing a healthy child. Such a decision may be based on one or more understandable factors. Perhaps the parents have not been clearly informed as to how the inheritance pattern might work; perhaps they have difficulty accepting it as reality for themselves and need to test it out; perhaps they have deep convictions that bearing children is the main purpose of sexuality and marriage. If their gamble is lost and the child afflicted, their self-reproach may be bitter.

Guilt Arising from Negative Feelings

The kindest and most conscientious parents have cause at times to feel irritation, disappointment, exasperation, resentment, or anger at their children. Parents of healthy children can usually accept these feelings and still feel adequate as parents. Parents of sick children tend to be more troubled by their negative feelings. In fact, when a sense of

*Patterns of inheritance are discussed in Chapter 8.

remorse or feelings of worthlessness persist and remain intense, it may well be that there are some unacknowledged angry feelings toward the child that need to be searched out and examined.

Perhaps a pregnancy was unplanned and untimely, and the baby's birth put an end to his mother's job or his father's hopes for a postgraduate degree. Even though the baby was appealing and received much devoted care, his parents may not have been able to dispel completely their resentment that he had disrupted their life scheme. If the baby was found to have a serious disorder, his parents would be likely to reproach themselves in misery: "Great people *we* are — couldn't think of anything but our own selfish plans. We wished sometimes we didn't have him. Now it looks as though our wish might even come true."

Perhaps a child, just before he became ill, had been in a particularly trying stage of development: negativistic, self-assertive, prone to outbursts of temper and of tears. There would have been many moments (especially on rainy, in-the-house days) when his mother wished for the power to banish him to Outer Mongolia. She could laugh at those thoughts — until he was hospitalized. Then she felt bitter remorse for her impatience and annoyance. She would have given anything — anything at all — to have one of those rainy days back, and to be shut in the house with a restless, irritable but healthy child.

Parents need to find satisfaction in child care, the sense of pride and accomplishment that grows out of observing one's child grow and gain and smile and take his first step — in his playpen, into the school bus. For many weeks (or even months or years), before anyone was sure what the trouble really was, your child may have been irritable and whiny and hard to live with. He may have been lethargic and seemed lazy, and moped around without doing anything worthwhile at all. He may have looked pale and puny. Perhaps he wasn't gaining or growing very much. He may have had an exasperating cough and a nose that never stopped running. You felt disappointed in him and worried about him and irritated at him all at once. Why should you have felt otherwise?

A nurse in a cystic fibrosis clinic commented on how alert, sociable, and responsive her new patient, Johnny, was at four months of age. "He acts like a baby who has had very good care," she complimented his parents. Johnny's mother flushed. Her quick glance toward her husband was troubled. "Well," she said, "I don't feel like a good mother. He would cry night after night after night. Jim and I had to take turns rocking him and walking him hour after hour. We were so tired all the time. There were moments when I couldn't stand Johnny any more — I felt like chucking him out of the window. Now I realize he was crying because he had gas and cramps in his tummy. Poor little fellow — I feel so mean and awful."

The feelings Johnny's mother described were closely related to a thought that is probably the most painful one of all for parents of sick children.

Mrs. O. was recounting to a group of other parents in the hospital how it had been when her baby, Margaret, had surgery for an intestinal blockage. "The doctor at home didn't know at first what the trouble was, so Margaret didn't have the operation soon enough. Day after day she was throwing up and crying — she must have been in pain. Hugh and I would sit by her in the hospital all day long, but we couldn't do anything for her." Mrs. O.'s face collapsed into the grimace of weeping. "You won't believe this — it sounds so awful to say — but Hugh and I, we actually began to hope that our own baby would die."

There was a rustle of movement around the table, and other parents were nodding in sympathy. "I used to think that I must be unnatural to feel that way," Mrs. S. said quietly, "but my husband, Alan, helped me to see that it really wasn't wicked at all. It was only a small part of what we have felt for Robert, and in a way it was a loving kind of feeling. Because what we really meant was this: We didn't mean that we wished him harm; what we meant was that rather than have him suffer we would wish him to be at peace."

Coming to Terms with Guilty Feelings

What are the steps that lead from self-accusation toward self-forgiveness? The first step — one of the hardest tasks facing you — is to search out within yourself the thoughts of being to blame for your child's illness and the feelings of remorse because your relationship with him was sometimes less than ideal. It may be almost unbearable to reflect about these ideas and feelings, let alone put them into words for another person to hear. This, however, is the next step. If you can gradually bring yourself to talk them over with someone you trust, it is likely that the intensity of your self-reproach will diminish. You may then be able to take the third step, namely, asking a doctor about the causes of your child's illness (in most cases he will reassure you that you were in no way to blame). Finally, you may need to make an effort to recognize all that has been positive in your care of your child and in your feelings about him. Perhaps you will then be able to accept that there are no human relationships altogether free of negative feelings, and will forgive yourself for your humanity.

If these steps are too difficult and you can't dispel your guilty feelings, it is likely that the help of a professional counselor is needed. Guilty feelings that persist often have their roots in the past and, like an infected cyst, may need to be opened gently and carefully and drained before healing can take place.

Anger

Throughout the natural world, adult creatures become fiercely aggressive when their young are in jeopardy. So may the human parent feel a surge of angry protest and, often, an impulse to fight when the human child is endangered. In nature, the adult can launch a direct attack — with fang, beak, or claw — on the agent of threat. But how does a human parent attack a diagnosis? How does he fight a disease? Where does he direct the feelings of anger?

Irritability in the Family

Sadly, those who care most about each other often use each other as targets of harsh and angry feelings. Parents in grief often describe an increase of irritable feelings toward each other.

Each may have critical or frankly hostile thoughts about the spouse. One parent may believe that the other was somehow to blame for the illness — through giving less than ideal care, through neglect or delay in seeking medical advice, or through carrying a particular genetic trait.

Often, the parent does not truly believe such accusatory thoughts. Rather, he feels profoundly disturbed and irritable, and seeks some justification for his hostility.

Parents may feel alienated from one another because they respond to anxiety and grief in quite different ways. The father, for example, may conceal his feelings stoically, and become more and more distant and aloof. He may be silent, absorbed in himself. He may seem coldly uncaring to the mother, who longs for closeness and tender sharing. Failing to sense the hidden anguish, she may resent him bitterly.

It may not be your spouse but another child in the family who becomes the target of your irritability, especially if the other child has reacted to the tension at home by becoming demanding and whiny. In fact, although you probably try to conceal this, you may have fleeting moments of resentment of your other children because they are so healthy. Why should they have all the joy of health and just one child have all the burden of illness?

In all such ways, the angry feelings — the need to fight — that have been aroused by your child's illness and that seek an outlet may be vented on those closest and most important to you.

Critical Feelings toward Doctors and Nurses

Some illnesses are difficult to diagnose. The early symptoms may be ones which could signify a number of different conditions. Diagnosis may require specialized medical procedures or laboratory tests which a family physician or local hospital are not equipped to perform. Therefore, diagnosis of your child's illness may have been delayed for weeks, months, even years. This period of delay would have resulted in prolonged apprehension and worry for you and your family, and perhaps in unrelieved misery for your child. At least one doctor may have dismissed your fears as groundless and termed you "overly anxious," making you uneasy about your own power of observation and judgment. Your medical expenses may have mounted alarmingly and to no avail. Although it is not always true that early diagnosis results in more effective treatment, it is understandable that you might have bitter feelings about the doctor or doctors who "missed the boat."

If your child has to be hospitalized, you may therefore find yourself feeling critical of almost everything done by the professional staff. The doctors may seem unavailable, hurried, brusque, more interested in lab reports than in your child's fears. The nurses may seem to convey a feeling that you are underfoot: "Your child is our patient now. We don't need you here." Without intending to, you may have blinded yourself to the actions that do reveal competence, concern, and compassion. (Sometimes, too, a doctor or nurse may be brusque to keep from crying.) In such ways, the anger aroused by your child's illness may be vented on the medical staff.

Bitterness toward the Church

Sometimes grieving parents lash out at their church, their God: "I've tried so hard to follow the teachings of my church, to be a good person, and now, this is my reward." "How can I go on believing in a God who could be so cruel, so punishing? I don't go to church any more." Thus religious faith — solace and source of strength for many people — may be weakened just at a time when it is desperately needed.

In relation to family, medical staff and church, justification for a parent's annoyance, irritability, bitterness, thoughts of blame can often be found. However, the underground river that feeds and reinforces such thoughts and feelings is the deep need to fight stirred by the child's illness. Until this need is recognized and given outlets, a parent may continue to vent his anger at any available target and, in so doing, damage relationships that could be sources of comfort and strength. A grieving parent needs family members, clergymen, doctors, and nurses to support him and to help his child.

Talking It Out

Talking it out is frequently advised and is frequently helpful in understanding and mastering troubled feelings. The value of verbal expression depends greatly, however, on the circumstances under which you ventilate, on the person chosen as the listener, and on the feelings to be expressed. Expressing angry feelings to the person you are angry at can be hazardous. Until there has been some opportunity to reflect a little about the anger and to relieve its intensity, angry words may become weapons of attack. They may stimulate counterattack; they may inflict wounds that are slow to heal; they may leave you feeling remorseful and wretched.

This is not to suggest that anger should be bottled up (to leak out in tone of voice, gesture, and facial expression). It may be helpful, though, to vent these explosive feelings first with an understanding and somewhat objective listener. After the intensity of the anger has been relieved by putting it in words, after you understand more clearly the source of the anger, then it can perhaps be expressed to the person you feel angry at, without attacking and wounding.

If a listener is not available, some of the anger might be released in writing. Write an angry letter, perhaps — but don't mail it until you have reviewed it the next day. An even better way to modulate anger and to discharge aggression is through bodily movement.

"Bodily Discharge"

In our technological society, the use of the human body for the discharge of aggression is inhibited. Women have, from girlhood, been discouraged in many subtle ways from physical activity. One hallmark of progress is considered to be the maximal substitution of electrical energy (through appliances) for muscular energy in housekeeping. Men have been encouraged to substitute passive and vicarious participation in sports (through TV viewing) for active involvement. Many jobs are carried out in a sitting position. Movement to and from the office or factory is often limited to the alternation of the right foot between car accelerator and brake (and this movement often becomes the most available and dangerous outlet for feelings of frustration and rage).

Bodily action, which the U.S. life-style tends to inhibit, can, however, be an immensely relieving and often constructive channel for the discharge of aggression. There are many possibilities in daily life for engaging the muscles in vigorous, even attacking movements. In the house, you may *scour* (the oven), *scrub* (the floor), *press* (kneading dough), *pound* (tenderizing meat or hammering nails). In the garden, you may *yank* (weeds), *hit* (with the hoe), *push* (a shovel or lawnmower). A variety of sports not only permit but actually require attack. You may *smash, wallop* or *fling* an object (playing golf, softball, squash, tennis, badminton, volley-ball, croquet, ping-pong, or bowling). You may *hurl* your own body (diving, jumping, running).

Other bodily activities are less aggressive but employ most of the large muscles in rhythmical, repetitive, and usually soothing motion: walking, skating, swimming, bicycle riding, for example. In addition to the relaxation engendered by the motion, activities such as these often place you in a relationship to nature that can be healing. A walk along the seashore, in a forest, or along a country road at night may introduce a new perspective: even the greatest of human anguish occupies only an infinitesimal portion of the universe.

Some of the activities suggested are familiar ones, although you may not have used them purposefully as outlets for your feelings. Others may be new, and may require trial before you can design a program that works for you. You may be reluctant to try at all. Intense emotion produces nervous and muscular tension that can result in deep fatigue. You may feel as though you have no energy for any unnecessary activity. But if you can induce yourself (or your family and friends can persuade you) to try such an outlet a few times, you may experience a renewal of energy. Discharge of the aggressive impulses that contribute to tension usually brings relaxation as well as an improved capacity to rest and to sleep.

Fighting for Your Child

"How does a human parent attack a diagnosis?" it was asked. "How does he fight a disease?" The aggressive drive, the wish to fight that may have been aroused by your child's illness can be directed toward a number of extremely significant goals of both direct and indirect benefit to your child and to others with similar needs. Since many of these goals will be considered in detail in later chapters, they will only be outlined here.

Parents can usefully fight by mastering the home-treatment program for the child (diet, medication, physical therapies) and by planning for future treatment needs (organizing donors to insure an ample supply of blood should transfusion be needed, for example). Parents can usefully fight by associating with others to educate the public about the particular disease (to promote better understanding of the needs of children such as theirs and to promote early diagnosis of the disorder), to raise funds for medical research and for medical equipment (such as that needed for inhalation therapy or hemodialysis at home). Parents can usefully fight by influencing hospital policies so that ample visiting of patients is allowed, so that facilities are made available for parents to room in with very young or very sick children, so that adequate play and educational programs are established for hospitalized children. Parents can usefully fight by influencing school policies regarding physical education programs, arrangements for taking medication, and accessibility of bathrooms for children with health problems. Parents can exert influence to modify the physical environment (schools, shops, theaters, museums so that accommodations are provided for those with health problems: ramps for those with limited stamina and shortness of breath; doorways wide enough to admit wheelchairs, for example. In these many ways, anger can become a constructive and significant force.

You may, at first, find it hard to imagine having the energy or motivation for such pursuits. But if you begin with a simple program of activity that releases some of your tension (a daily walk, half an hour at the piano), you may experience a surprising renewal of energy.

Apprehension and Anxiety

Am I Normal?

"How do other parents feel at a time like this? How do they behave?" It is not likely that these questions would be raised in a Greek mountain community, an Irish village — in any ethnic group in which grief is openly expressed, shared, and accepted as an inescapable part of human existence. Here, however, these questions are frequently asked by grieving parents who feel anxious about their reactions, feelings, and behavior and wonder, "Am I normal?"

The mother of a toddler hospitalized with a kidney disease complained, "I can't get my housework done — I can't get anything done — I just sit around the apartment all day doing nothing. I just sit." Another parent, usually efficient and well organized, was frightened to find, after coming home from marketing and putting the groceries away, that she had put a packet of light bulbs in the refrigerator and the butter in the broom closet. (Her concern was particularly intense because her own mother had once undergone psychiatric hospitalization, and she had long feared that there might be some hereditary mental instability in the family.) The father of a teenage girl with a recently diagnosed blood disease mourned, "I used to be a happy man. Now I walk the floor every night. I can't think, I can't make decisions, I don't know what's right. I feel as though my brain is in a plastic bag." Mrs. W. found herself screaming at people, even hurling dishes around the kitchen, and she feared that she might injure her children in one of her angry outbursts.

For these parents, the intense emotions or the changed mental or behavioral state — apathy, confusion, disorganization, forgetfulness, indecisiveness, loss of control — were frightening and aroused the questions, "Am I normal?" "Am I losing my mind?" For other parents, the most urgent questions may be, "What lies ahead?" "Will I be able to bear it?" "Will I have a breakdown?" Mrs. B. was rigidly controlled each time she visited her child in the hospital. Her visits were brief, and she made obvious attempts to avoid contact with the staff or other parents. One day, when she was trembling visibly, a nurse expressed concern. Mrs. B. then described her fear that she might start to cry and if she began, she would weep and weep and weep, and never be able to stop.

Am I Alone?

Mrs. B. overlooked the fact that there would be people standing by, people to comfort her and to help her stop crying. This was readily overlooked because grief is isolating; you feel alone, and to be so alone is frightening. You may feel alone because you and close family members have turned away from each other to deal with your distress in privacy before you can turn back and offer solace or receive it. You may feel alone because of a sense of alienation from friends and relatives. (How, you wonder, could anyone who has never experienced such grief understand what it is like?) You may feel alone because your resentment and anger about your child's illness has kept at a distance the minister, nurse, or doctor who could help. You may feel alone because, even in the closest family, there are vulnerable moments. At night, for example, after your husband or wife has fallen asleep you may become lost in a solitary, grief-filled reverie. There is nobody to hear your fears, no reality against which to measure your fancies; there are no boundaries to your despair.

Am I sick, Too?

Close and tender as the relationship between father and child may be, it still lacks the biological attachment that develops between mother and infant through the long months of pregnancy and that may continue through a period of breast-feeding. And after biological separation has occurred, the care of an infant still involves close bodily contact and intimacy. Even in our changing society, with its shifts in the roles of parents, such intimate care is usually provided by the mother. Understandably, then, some mothers feel a special sense of attachment to the child that is different from the bond between father and child: "The child is of my flesh and blood, a part of myself." To a mother with such feelings, danger to the child can also seem as danger to herself. Perhaps this is why mothers in grief may (more readily than fathers) become fearful about the well-being of their own bodies.

The human body responds to emotional stress with physiological change. A pounding heart, breathlessness, trembling and perspiring hands, pallor, dry mouth, frog-in-the-throat, digestive upsets and frequent urination are among the many common bodily expressions of fear, anger, or sorrow. How easy it becomes for a grieving, deeply worried mother to wonder if a disease in her own body is causing these disturbing physical sensations. Is the sharp pain in her chest from stomach spasm, or is it a heart attack? Is the change in her menstrual rhythm caused by tension, or is it a sign of cancer? These are frightening questions that can occupy the mind and bring terror, especially in lonely moments.

Can I Safeguard My Child?

The sense of helplessness that may be aroused when your child becomes ill is frightening. The illness is a threat to his safety that seems largely beyond your control. True, all children, all people, are to some extent at risk. A child cannot be totally protected. He may be knocked off his bike by a car, he may blow his mind with LSD, he may have to go to war. But parents of healthy children can, and do, console themselves with denial: "That won't happen to *my* child." Such consolation has been brutally stripped away from you. You may feel overwhelmed by the fear that no matter what you do or how you do it, it won't be enough.

On the other hand, and just as frightening, you may feel certain that the life of your child is *altogether* in your hands. It will be up to you to carry out his treatments, give his medicine, balance his diet, regulate his activity, protect him from infection. How, you wonder, can you possibly know enough, be wise enough, skillful enough, protective enough? What if you make a mistake, use poor judgment, hurt your child, cause him serious harm? The family wage earner may wonder, "Can I provide well enough to meet his medical needs? What if I don't get promoted? What if I lose my job?"

So it is equally frightening to feel you can do nothing and to feel you must do everything for your child. Neither expectation is realistic, but only gradually will you develop confidence in your capacity to help your child; only gradually will you accept that there are limitations on what you can reasonably expect of yourself; only gradually will you become aware that you are a member of a team working on his behalf.

Mastering Anxiety

Although some components of your grief reaction, guilt, for example, can be dispelled to a large extent, anxiety and apprehension about your child tend to become woven into the fabric of daily life. They may be aroused by routine observations or events: the sound of your child's cough, the impression that he looks pale, a visit to the doctor for a checkup, hospitalization for a transfusion or a special medication. Apprehension and anxiety can be mastered, perhaps through the following measures. And mastery in the early stages of your child's illness can pave the way for mastery of feelings that develop later.

Examining Fears.   Examine your fears — those about yourself and those about your child. The ideas concealed in a secret part of your mind that slip loose in solitude or darkness are often cloaked in dread and horror. But what you imagine is usually much more fearsome than the reality. For this reason, it is most important to bring your fears out into the daylight and talk them over with someone who is competent to help you sort them out. Some fears will be promptly dispelled in the light of reality; it will be obvious to you that they are unfounded. Others may need to be examined even further with persons qualified to give particular information. Only your own doctor, for example, can alleviate your fear that your chest pain might be a symptom of heart disease.

Modifying Expectations.   Within your family and at your job, there are needs that must be met and people that must be responded to. However, it is not reasonable to expect yourself to function in times of grief as you would in normal times. (Would you expect this if you had influenza? Grief can be just as disabling.) If you ask too much of yourself, your reduced capacity to perform may increase your anxiety. On the other hand, it is not helpful to ask too little of yourself, even though you may long to be free of responsibility and let others care for you. If you ask little of yourself, and encourage those around to ask little of you, there is risk that each day may become a void in which the only reality is the anguish absorbing you — and who can bear that much pain? There is risk that you will reproach yourself for neglecting those who need you, and that your emotional burden will be thus increased.

Using All Available Support. Work is a support because it is organizing and healing. It gives form and structure to the day; it gives some sense of accomplishment and self-satisfaction; it offers channels for discharge of tension. A wage earner, unless he stays away from the job, is impelled to function by the expectations of those he works with and for. A homemaker must shape each day herself, often relying on spontaneous judgments to decide which tasks should be given priority, which set aside. In a time of grief, it may be useful to develop a simple but definite program for the day. With the help of a relative, friend, or neighbor, determine which needs you must meet and when you must meet them. A written schedule may be a useful aid; a mechanical timer might be organizing while the tasks are being carried out. Try to deal with one small segment of reality at a time (for example, your child's need for clean pajamas). Since there may be many tasks you feel unable to cope with, it is wise to accept help from any available source, including friendly assistance from neighbors and paid services. Your need is legitimate and probably only temporary since your usual level of functioning will gradually be restored.

It is important also to seek every aid to physical well-being: a long walk to relieve your nervousness and agitation, a warm bath or a glass of wine to ease your sleeplessness, a favorite food to coax back your appetite. If such aids fail to offer sufficient relief, it is important to consult your doctor about the temporary use of medication, perhaps a sedative or tranquilizer. (If you attempt to dose yourself without his advice, you may increase the very condition you are attempting to relieve. Certain tranquilizers, for example, are known to intensify feelings of depression.) A state of physical exhaustion will not help you master your grief, nor will it enable you to help your ill child.

Considering Professional Help. There are many ways professionally trained persons can help you meet the challenge of your child's illness; the contributions of doctors, nurses, social workers, clergymen, physiotherapists, and others are discussed frequently in this book. In regard to fears about yourself, there are some signals that indicate the help of a mental health professional is needed.

First, it is wise to keep in mind that each parent facing the crisis of a potentially serious disorder in his child tends to respond in an individual way. The intensity of a parent's feelings and his pace in recognizing these feelings vary in accord with personality and past experience.

Mrs. R. became profoundly depressed when her infant daughter was found to have an intestinal disorder resulting in cramping pain, diarrhea, and failure to thrive. Although the baby's doctor expected that the disorder would be controlled by a special diet and medication, Mrs. R.'s sadness, apprehension, and self-reproach were not relieved.

As Mrs. R. discussed her feelings with a professional social worker, she began to remember her earlier years when her mother had had a chronic diarrhea — and later developed a cancer from which she died. The illness of Mrs. R.'s baby (totally different from that of her mother, except that both produced diarrhea) had revived her grief and her forgotten feelings of blame for her mother's illness. Her despair about her baby was unrealistic, but could not be dispelled until she worked out the tangled web of her unfinished mourning of her mother's death.

In Mrs. R.'s case, a grief reaction in the present was greatly complicated by a grief experience in the past. It was the fact that her reaction to her baby's illness was more intense and pessimistic than the baby's condition warranted that signaled her need for professional help.

There are other types of indications also. For example, anxiety sometimes becomes disabling — that is, it renders a person unable to function in essential ways. Occasionally, a parent may experience panic states in which he finds it impossible to stay in the house alone or to drive a car. Occasionally, a parent may develop severe and painful physical symptoms that the doctor believes are caused by emotional distress. Occasionally, a parent may feel such despair that he can see no solution other than suicide. Occasionally, a parent may feel that his controls are slipping dangerously and there is a risk that he will hurt a child in anger. In any such instances, it is wise to seek the advice of a psychiatrist in determining whether psychotherapy, medication, or supportive help would be most useful.

Gathering Information about the Tasks Ahead. A central task is to understand and learn to cope with the powerful emotions that have been described. These feelings will be aroused again and again as you deal with your child's health impairment. The more honestly you can recognize them, and the more constructively you can express them, the more effectively will you master the challenges facing you.

Your child's disorder will influence every relationship within your family. The other children will at times need special consideration, and they will need your help in understanding and accepting the claims of their ill sibling. Your marriage will at times need special consideration, since strains arising from a child's health impairment can either erode or strengthen the conjugal bonds. A parent who is single will need to find outside support and solace.

The attitudes of parents are more significant than the severity of the illness in determining how effectively a child copes with impaired health. In each phase of his development, medical problems have special meaning for a child and for his parents. In each phase, new concerns will arise. If these are recognized, many problems can be avoided. It is within your power as a parent to help your afflicted child develop his capabilities as fully as possible, develop meaningful relationships to others, and learn to value himself as a human being.

The remainder of this book is devoted to discussion of these complex challenges that you face. It is also devoted to discussion of the many and varied solutions that children, their families, and professional people have found to be helpful in meeting the challenges.

2

Safeguarding Family Relationships

Your Marriage

Parents who face the threat of their child's illness or disability — and their own fear of loss — need the comfort of closeness and human warmth. Ironically, it is at just such a time that their marriage becomes vulnerable. The threat to their child, rather than drawing them together, can alienate them. The closest, most devoted couples may sense the strain; others may feel like hostile strangers.

Who's to Blame?

The sense of angry protest that parents of sick children experience seeks a target. The most available target is usually one's husband or wife. Parents may, therefore, engage in angry, even bitter accusations of each other that can leave deep wounds in their relationship.

Blame for Inheritance. The husband or wife is readily blamed for carrying the "bad seed" that caused an inherited illness. Relatives who can't endure the idea that their family lineage is somehow "tainted" may reinforce the accusations: "It must be her side of the family — it certainly couldn't be ours."

Such blame may bear little relationship to reality. For example, hemophilia is transmitted *by* the female *to* the male (page 209). One might suppose that fathers of hemophiliac sons would find it difficult to forgive their wives for passing on the illness. A few do. The majority, however, soon recognize that the responsibility for the pregnancy was shared, and therefore the responsibility for the outcome was shared. In contrast, a disorder such as cystic fibrosis is passed by *both* parents (page 208). Even knowing this, one spouse may gather elaborate information to show that "there have been several cases on his side of the family and none on mine — therefore it obviously comes *more* from his side than from mine!"

Blame for "Neglect." No parent can provide what the other might consider ideal care of a child all of the time. Therefore, one parent can usually recall some event which may seem (usually mistakenly) to have contributed to the illness.

Jerry's father adored his only son (Chapter 1). When Jerry's encephalitis developed, he might readily have turned his bitterness against his wife: "You *knew* he had a cold, you *knew* he's clumsy when he gets excited, you *knew* he would have to cross that stream to get to the lake! Why on earth did you let him go?"

Blame for Delay in Seeing the Doctor. In many families, one parent becomes worried about a child's health sooner than the other. The other may ignore the fears or scoff at them, so that consultation with the child's doctor is delayed.

When Priscilla was found to have leukemia, her mother could scarcely stop berating her husband: "I *told* you she wasn't right. I *told* you she was sickening — getting pale and listless, tired all the time. You wouldn't listen, would you? Told me I was just a worrywart, didn't you? I didn't know what was the right thing to do. If you'd let me take her to the doctor right off, maybe he could have done more for her."

Differences in Coping Style

Parents may each react to grief and worry in a different way. A wife may seek to share her feelings, to express them in words, and perhaps in tears, to seek physical intimacy with her husband, hoping he will hold her close and comfort her. Instead of coming closer, her husband may seem to retreat, to become more silent and aloof. He may try to bury his pain under an avalanche of work, spending more and more time at his job, perhaps accepting special assignments that will increase his income and keep him away from home. The wife may feel dejected and disappointed: "He doesn't care about me any more." The husband may feel unable to endure her tears because he fears that he will lose control of his own.

On the other hand, the wife may herself withdraw into her grief. Sad and weary, she may be unable to do more than keep the family fed and clothed. At every opportunity, she may retreat from her pain by taking a nap. She may seem uncaring of the needs and feelings of those around her. Her husband can readily feel, "She doesn't care about me any more."

Parents who are fully sensitive to each other's emotions may play a game of "I'll hide my feelings so that you won't realize how worried I am." Such parents hope that if they conceal their own fears, the spouse will find it easier to sustain hope; they hope that the spouse will conclude, "If he isn't worried, it can't really be serious."

In any such case, the privacy of one partner may leave the other feeling abandoned. Rather than drawing closer to share their grief, husband and wife become strangers. The burden of worry about the child is cruelly magnified by their loss of sharing and of trust.

Doesn't My Child Need Me?

In our society, it is still usually the mother who assumes the major care-taking role for the child, and, thus, the central responsibility for meeting the needs of an ill child. The traditional system of communication about the ill child usually involves doctor-*mother*-child. For both these reasons, father is often excluded from a meaningful role in the child's care. For many men, this situation adds to existing feelings of helplessness about the illness. It may spur the father to spend still *more* time on the job so that he can provide at least financially for the child's care. As the mother's absorption in the ill child increases, as the father attempts desperately to play a useful part outside the home, the emotional distance between husband and wife becomes even greater.

The risk of such a development is increased if the mother had a particularly close relationship with the child before the illness. (There are certain stages in a child's development when one parent and the child may form a special alliance that seems to close out the other parent.)

Peter was four when he developed nephrosis. For a year or more, he and his mother had felt a specially tender attachment to each other. Peter often declared his intention of marrying his mother later on, and supporting her in luxurious style from his earnings as a jet pilot. Understandably, if not altogether wisely, Peter's mother basked in the sunshine of his devotion (which went far to compensate for some dissatisfactions in her marriage); she gave subtle approval and encouragement to Peter's possessiveness, and to his attempts to keep his father from coming close to her.

When Peter became ill, his mother tried to meet *every* need and fulfill *every* wish herself. When he was hospitalized, she was distraught. She declared herself unable to go home until Peter could go too. His toys would be strewn around. In particular, she couldn't bear to see his bedroom. The house would be bleak, empty.

Peter's father stood listening to her dejectedly. The droop of his head and his sagging shoulders suggested his despair. Finally he looked up and reached a hand toward his wife: "You still have me, dear." She shook her head and turned away. Her husband went home alone.

Changes in Life-style

Every family has its own particular style of living. A child's illness may result in significant changes. In some instances, the family may have to move. For example, it may be unwise for a child with severe heart disease to live at a high altitude. A child with cystic fibrosis may need to live reasonably close to a major medical center. The chief wage earner in a family may decide to seek a different job that offers a higher income or greater possibility for advancement in order to meet the costs of medical care.

The pattern of leisure-time activities may be altered. There may, for example, be less time available for shared recreation; some favorite activities may have to be curtailed because of their expense.

Just at this time, when husband and wife most need to come together and share deeply with each other, there may be interference in their sexual relationship. Either or both may feel exhausted, physically or emotionally. The needs of the ill child may reduce the amount of time available to them for intimate solitude. They may feel apprehensive about the possibility of another pregnancy.

Impaired Communication

For any or all of the reasons described, the marital relationship is subject to strain. One of the most serious results of such strain may be a breakdown in constructive communication. Temporarily alienated from each other, sharing space and food but not thoughts or feelings, husband and wife can become virtual strangers. Understanding little of the actual meaning of the child's illness to the marital partner, each may *imagine* what the other feels, often misinterpreting the clues badly.

When she was three and a half, Paula's relationship with her mother was a typical mixed blessing. At moments, Paula was affectionate, happily "helped" her mother with the housework, and declared her wish to be "just like Mommy" when she grew up. Just as often, she was disobedient and impudent. Showing the tender adoration of her father that Peter had shown to his mother, Paula boisterously asserted her claims to her father's attention and treated her mother as though she were an unwelcome rival. Like many mothers of such daughters, Paula's mother vacillated between affection and annoyance. By the end of the afternoon, when her husband came home, it was usually the annoyance that predominated. This was the feeling most evident to Paula's father.

When Paula developed severe diabetes, with a sudden and frightening onset, Paula's mother felt tormented. She reproached herself for every outburst of irritability toward the child, realizing how deeply she cared about her daughter. Absorbed in her own unhappiness, she was only partially aware of her husband's critical attitude and his growing hostility toward her.

To the hospital staff both parents appeared irritable, fault-finding and uncommunicative. It was decided that the social worker would let the couple know of the staff's concern, and help them explore the sources of difficulty.

In a conference between Paula's parents and the social worker, the misery underlying their hostile demeanor was quickly revealed. Having observed primarily the moments of irritability and rivalry between his wife and daughter, Mr. R. had wrongly concluded that his wife cared little for his beloved child. This conclusion had aroused enormous resentment now that Paula was so ill. Mrs. R., responding to the resentment she sensed in him, retreated more deeply into her own remorse. She felt so defensive that almost any human contact struck sparks of irritability.

A child's illness does not inevitably destroy the parents' marriage. To the contrary, among a group of families of children with cystic fibrosis, it was found that the divorce rate was lower than in the general population. However, the period of coming to terms with the illness is one of severe strain in most marriages. Most, perhaps all couples would benefit from an opportunity to explore together their thoughts and feelings with a listener able to be objective, accepting, and understanding. Couples who are able to establish, or reestablish, bridges of communication in a time of such stress often find that they develop emotional bonds of great depth and enduring strength.

Your Other Children

What Is Wrong?

Parents facing a serious health problem in their child often wonder, "Should I tell the other children?" There is, realistically, no alternative to telling them, since the children will soon become aware that *something* is wrong. Your facial expression, your tone of voice, the way you carry your body — perhaps a slowness in responding to them or an unusual irritability — all these are signals of trouble. Sensing trouble without knowing its source is extremely worrying for children.

Without some realistic information, your children will supply their own interpretations of all that they see, hear, and sense. These interpretations may be distorted and more frightening than the truth. For example, scenes in which emergency help must be given to a sick child (perhaps to relieve an asthmatic attack or a convulsion) are easily misconstrued. Siblings — brothers and sisters — sometimes believe that the adults, in their swift, excited actions, are attacking and hurting the ill child and causing rather than relieving his distress.

The choice, therefore, is scarcely *whether* to tell but, rather, *how* and *what* to tell. Many parents worry that they won't be able to discuss their child's illness without showing emotion. They fear, in particular, that they may break down and weep. This can indeed happen. Why, though, should it harm your children to know that you have feelings, especially if you can express them honestly?: "I do feel sad because Jimmy is sick. Sometimes it makes me sad enough to cry." Such a moment of shared sorrow (in which your child may try to comfort you) can be one of special and tender closeness. It may show your children that it is all right for them, also, to express feelings and to talk about them.

A prolonged, intense, and uncontrolled expression of your grief could be worrying for them. Therefore, it may be easier for you and for them if you talk about the illness while carrying on some buffering activity — taking a walk together, raking the lawn, making the beds. The movement will help to relieve some of the tension in the discussion. Your children may also, as you talk, seek comfort from their own bodies — a young girl may suck her thumb or twist a lock of hair, a little boy may reach anxiously at his penis.

You might begin the conversation with the simple statement that the doctor has told you your child has an illness. You might then encourage the child's brother or sister to express his own ideas and concerns by saying: "You must wonder why Paul has to stay in the hospital." "You must wonder why Jennie has been so tired and cranky." "You must wonder what makes Billy cough so much." It is wise not to force information on your children, but to explain that you will try to answer their questions when they are ready to ask. This goes far to establish a climate of trust. The information you give will need to be repeated many times. As your children develop, their ideas and attitudes will change; as your ill child develops, his condition and his needs will change. Should you feel unable to deal with a question, it is all right to postpone answering it ("Jane, you've caught me at a bad moment when I'm very busy and tired; I'd like to talk with you about that later on") or to arrange for your child to talk with a doctor or nurse about it ("I don't know how to answer that question, but you do need an answer. Let's see if you could talk it over with Dr. Brown").

Some parents fear that if there is any discussion of the illness, the questions will lead inexorably toward the most dreaded one: "Is Jerry going to die?" Other parents are reluctant to name an illness such as cystic fibrosis, Cooley's anemia, or leukemia, knowing that their children may then read or be told frightening things about these disorders. To dread questions about your ill child's future is understandable, since these questions force you to face your deepest fears. At some time, however, such questions will need to be discussed. If your children cannot find answers from you, they will seek them elsewhere.

What might you tell the child who asks, "Is my brother going to die?" Some parents are able to tell the truth if it is worded somewhat like this: "I can't give you an absolutely certain answer" (parents with religious beliefs may add, "Only God knows how long people will live"). "It's true that right now the doctors don't know how to make Jerry completely well again. There is a lot they can do to make him feel better, though. They are learning more about his illness every day. We hope that they will soon discover how to make him healthy again." Should your eyes fill with tears, should your voice quaver, you might add, "I do feel sad about Jerry. I wish he were healthy again right now."

Painful as such questions are for you, for your children there are others that are also extremely urgent. Whether or not these questions are put directly into words, they are almost certain to occupy the thoughts of your children at some time.

Is It My Fault?

Brothers and sisters are allies, rivals, protectors, scapegoats, leaders, followers, devoted friends, and bitter enemies. They feel love, hate, jealousy, admiration, loyalty, and resentment toward each other. In every sibling relationship (as in every meaningful human relationship), there is some negative element, some trace of hostility.

Children have limited understanding of the connections between cause and effect. When puzzled, they tend to supply their own theories of causality, untroubled as to whether the theories are logical or realistic. At the same time, they often imagine their own thoughts and wishes to be powerful indeed. Therefore, if a child has had a hostile thought about his brother, and something bad (illness, for example) then happens to his brother, he may readily conclude that it is the result of his "bad" thought. It is commonly found that siblings of an ill child do anxiously wonder "Is it my fault?" even though they may not be able to put the question into words.

Furthermore, distraught parents sometimes contribute to a sibling's sense of responsibility.

As a baby, Penny had a narrow escape from the poorly understood illness often termed "accidental crib death." While in the kitchen with her mother and three-year-old brother, Penny suddenly made a faint choking sound and slumped down in her infant seat, no longer breathing. As her mother darted toward her, she snapped accusingly at her son, "What did you put in her mouth?" By her frantic efforts, Penny's mother revived the baby from what doctors later believed to have been a momentary cardiac arrest. Penny's brother had put nothing in her mouth, and his mother reassured him many times that she had made a mistake in blaming him. Had Penny not recovered, however, her brother and mother might for many years have shared in misery the thought that he had somehow caused her death.

Mike's parents wondered, when he developed encephalitis, an inflammation of the brain, whether his sister might have caused it because she had frequently played a game of "bump heads" with the baby. Parents of children with cystic fibrosis frequently caution their other children when they develop colds, "Don't get too close to Howard — he'll catch your cold." If Howard does develop a cold, and especially if a more serious respiratory infection follows, a brother or sister can easily feel responsible.

It is, therefore, important for parents to remember how easily their healthy children may come to feel responsible for the ill child's disorder. Your healthy children need direct reassurance just as much as you needed to know that you were not responsible for your child's disorder.

Children who accept reassurance that their sibling's illness was not a result of their own wishes, thoughts, or deeds may still feel guilty because they have moments of anger toward the ill child or resentment about the attention he is given. It is relieving if you can explain that you understand the resentment and that it is all right — not wicked — for the child to feel that way at times.

Guilt, it has been pointed out, is among the most tormenting of emotions. People who feel persistently guilty tend to seek ways to expiate or atone for their guilt. Children do this through seeking punishment in various ways: they may misbehave repeatedly, take obvious physical risks, have frequent accidents, fail in school, withdraw from friends and activities they had enjoyed. Should your children begin to show such behavior, it would be wise to evaluate the situation with a professional person.

Could It Happen to Me, Too?

Because of his close attachment to the ill child, because of his lack of understanding of the cause of the illness, or because he expects retribution for his own "bad" thoughts or feelings, your healthy child will probably wonder whether the same fate is to befall him. This question, also, may be expressed only in indirect ways: "By the way, what makes a person get a sick kidney?" It may not be asked at all, but be revealed through increased concern about his own bodily functions and sensations — his bruises, sniffles, coughs, and pains.

Quite unintentionally, you may increase his concern if you feel apprehensive about him. If your ill child has an inherited disorder such as cystic fibrosis, you may worry that your other children are affected also but feel unable to face having the diagnostic test ("sweat test") done to rule it out. If your ill child has an acquired illness, such as nephrosis or leukemia, your other children may now seem almost unbearably precious, and you may have become protective and restrictive toward them. Sensing this, the children may begin to feel vulnerable.

Your children will need realistic and repeated reassurance about themselves. Your family doctor or pediatrician may be helpful in this respect. Acquired illnesses of a serious nature are, after all, rare indeed within the total population. Many inherited disorders can be ruled out by special tests.

If brothers and sisters do possibly carry a genetic trait that might result in an inherited disorder's being passed on to their offspring, they should have the benefit of genetic education and counseling (Chapter 8). This source of help is likely to be most useful and meaningful during adolescence.

Don't You Care about Me?

Unavoidably, your relationship with your healthy children will be influenced by their sibling's illness. There will be changes in your mood — times of sadness when you are unable to share their joys and triumphs; moments of irritability when you snap at them and scold them unreasonably. There will be times when you seem remote and unresponsive, absorbed in your own thoughts and unaware of theirs. Alternately, you may hover over your healthy children with intense concern and protectiveness. You may feel flashes of resentment — why should your sick child have all the misery and your other children all the health? When you have three sons, why did your only daughter have to be the one to get sick?

You will need to give special attention to your ill child, carry out his treatment, take him to the doctor, be with him in the hospital. The needs of other children may sometimes have to take second place, even if they are too young to understand what is happening.

During his babyhood, Charlie suffered from a life-threatening allergic reaction to a particular group of foods. Whenever he became acutely ill, it was essential for his mother to take him to the hospital as rapidly as possible. She would leave his two-year-old brother, Scott, in the care of any available neighbor until her husband could return home.

During the sudden absences of Charlie and his mother, Scott would wander from room to room, as though searching. Desolately, he would ask, "Where Mommy gone? Where Baby gone?" After each separation experience, he would cling anxiously to his mother for many weeks, protesting even her brief, private visits to the bathroom.

Children readily give their own interpretation to your changes of mood, withdrawal of attention, and actual absences. Too readily, they may conclude that you have lost interest in them, stopped loving them, and that this must be because they are not lovable. They can scarcely avoid feeling resentful of the child who seems favored; they may attempt to claim their share of attention by acting babyish or by becoming ill themselves (in young children, emotional distress is readily transformed into physical ailments).

Forthright expression of your feelings and encouragement of your child in expressing his own can be helpful in preventing a buildup of distress. It can be relieving to both if you can say, "I'm sorry, Allen, I'm feeling tired and crabby today. I care about you very much, you know, but I've had to do a lot for Judy," or, "I know it makes you feel disappointed and angry that you have to miss baseball practice because of Judy's doctor's appointment. I understand your feeling. I feel very bad about it, too." Siblings need also to know that there are acceptable outlets for their angry and resentful feelings. For example, the siblings of a child with hemophilia or osteogenesis imperfecta can learn that although physical attacks on the ill child are forbidden, they may whack a punching bag or kick a ball until their fury is spent. It's all right, too, to shout, "You creep, you make me sooooooo mad!"

Parents are understandably shocked if they hear a brother or sister shout, usually in anger, a wish that the ill child will die: "I'm glad you have cystic fibrosis, Eve. I hope you'll die pretty soon," or, "Never mind, Ken, you're going to be with the angels next year!" Such utterances do burst out. They are likely to represent an explosion of resentment that has been building up over some time. But they may also reflect fear. "I hope you're going to die" is an indirect way of asking, "Are you really going to die?"

Parents, understandably, are inclined to respond with a reproach: "What an awful thing to say!" More helpful — although difficult — would be to say something of this sort: "It upsets me to hear that. I know there are moments when you're angry at Jack and you wish he weren't here. But that's only part of what you feel. At moments you care about him very much, and at times I imagine you worry about him. Are you feeling bothered now?"

Parents sometimes try to reduce their children's feelings of being neglected and their resentment by encouraging them to assume a helping role toward the sick child. Siblings of a child with hemophilia can monitor his play, cautioning him against climbing the weak limb of a tree and discouraging physical roughness among his playmates. Siblings of a child with cystic fibrosis can read him a story while postural drainage is being done and help the parent assemble the equipment for inhalation therapy. Siblings of a child with nephrosis can agree to eat their salty potato chips away from the house.

In many such ways, siblings can participate in the care of the ill child, and gain a sense of accomplishment as well as a feeling of being included. But it is most important to make certain that the brother or sister doesn't feel that the welfare (or the life) of the ill child is in his hands. He needs to know that at times things may go wrong in spite of the medical treatment.

It would be unfortunate if your healthy son did have to miss his baseball practice again and again because of Judy's doctor's appointments. There will be many times when the help of neighbors, friends, and relatives will be needed. People who care about you will be pleased if you suggest a useful role for them, which might well include seeing that your son does get to baseball.

Grief Reactions in Siblings

In households beset with grief and anxiety, the healthy children sometimes appear indifferent or uncaring. Their responses can be puzzling to adults and arouse resentment: "Children are heartless, cruel." Children do, of course, feel intense sorrow, apprehension, anger, and guilt, but they are not able to experience these feelings as you experience them nor respond to them as you do. The immature personality cannot endure a sustained awareness of emotional pain. There is only a short "sadness span."

Brothers and sisters of your ill child may show feelings that are the reverse of what you would expect. They may act silly, play the clown, fool around, laugh uproariously (often more in tense excitement than in joy). They may deny that your ill child has anything wrong with him at all or that they are at all bothered because he is sick.

Observing your own sadness and worry, siblings may feel uncomfortable because they don't feel the same. It is helpful to let them know that you don't expect them to — you know they can't. It is also helpful to be alert to signs that buried emotions are finding indirect expression.

Diana was eight when her brother, Jamie, was hospitalized for the third time. Afflicted with cystic fibrosis, Jamie had developed pneumonia. Although each hospitalization had been keenly worrisome for the family, the regimen of special drugs and intensive inhalation therapy had resulted in improvement. There was no reason to believe that the outcome would be different this time.

Diana showed no unusual worry about Jamie. However, when the time came to get ready for Sunday school, Diana began to feel sick to her stomach, and tearfully begged to stay home. This was repeated the following week.

Diana's mother, a particularly thoughtful and perceptive young woman, expressed concern about this to a social worker during her next visit to Jamie in the hospital. As they reviewed the problem together, Mrs. M. recalled that the Sunday school class had recently begun discussing the concepts of death and of life-after-death. These subjects had been introduced just before Jamie's hospitalization. It seemed, therefore, that Sunday school had become a ready outlet through which Diana's underlying anxiety about Jamie could be indirectly expressed. Her attempt to avoid Sunday school was her response to the anxiety.

It was decided that Mrs. M. would encourage Diana to express her questions and concerns about Jamie directly. As this began to occur, Diana's avoidance symptoms at first diminished and then disappeared.

Whenever there is a marked change in the mood, behavior, or accomplishments of your children, it may be helpful to consider (with a professional person if possible) what role the illness of your one child may be playing in the lives of the others.

Grandparents

Facing their child's illness, dealing with the strains this imposes on their marriage, meeting the needs of their other children, parents themselves need understanding and comfort. It is natural for them to wish for someone wise and strong to depend on, to wish that their own parents could offer the needed emotional support. Unfortunately, many parents of ill children find that their own parents cannot, particularly at first, be very helpful. In fact, grandparents may show typical responses that are very unhelpful indeed.

Typical Responses

Grandparents may steadfastly deny that your child could possibly have a medical disorder. They may express stronger doubts and more lasting disbelief than you, the child's own parents. They may repeatedly stir up or intensify your own uncertainty about whether you have done the best thing for your child. They may stir up or intensify your own secret doubts about whether your child's doctor is right. The disbelief of your parents can interfere badly with your own struggle to come to terms with the truth.

Grandparents may seem unable to understand what you tell them about your child's condition; they may become confused, forget significant facts. They may then besiege you with questions so that you must go over the painful story again and again.

Grandparents may become so upset, even distraught, that there is a reversal of roles. They do not comfort you; to the contrary, you find yourself trying to comfort them. At a time when you are struggling to muster every shred of courage and hope, your parents' displays of distress may weaken your own controls and drain your own emotional resources.

Grandparents — particularly if they grew up in another country, a different culture — may have a system of values and beliefs different from your own. They may expect from you certain kinds of behavior that you do not find helpful. For example, they may expect you to appear constantly grief stricken; they may expect you to give up all outside activities during a time when recreation and contact with your friends is essential in relieving your worry and sadness for brief moments.

In each of these ways, your parents may increase your emotional burden rather than sharing it. Their responses may leave you feeling hurt, disappointed, resentful, angry. Neither you nor your parents would wish it to be this way; they as much as you would probably wish that they could feel genuine compassion — a sensitive understanding of your feelings and a sensitive response to your needs. Unfortunately, such compassion is difficult for them to attain.

Barriers to Compassion

Whatever their outward attitudes may be, it is likely that your parents care deeply about you and your child. For this reason, both the reality of his illness and the intensity of your distress may be too painful for them to face.

If the disorder is an inherited one, their sense of responsibility may be as keen as your own but their understanding much less enlightened. Within their system of beliefs, inherited disorders may still be viewed as a taint in the family lineage and a source of shame.

Your parents may have arrived at a period in their own lives in which they have been struggling to face painful realities about themselves: the approach of the change of life; a decline in physical stamina and endurance; troubling questions about their accomplishments in their work and their future after retirement. They may not have the emotional resources available to meet your needs as they would wish.

Finally, as you grew through adolescence into adulthood, you probably communicated (loudly and strongly) your own wish for independence from your parents. Even when your need for comfort and support is intense, you may find it very difficult to reverse this trend of communication and to let them know clearly, "I need you now."

For any of these reasons, it may be difficult for a while to communicate with your parents about your child's health problem. Rather than giving repeated explanations, you may prefer to offer them a pamphlet about the disorder or to arrange for them to have a conference with your child's doctor. Rather than listening too often to their expressions of sorrow and worry, you may need to encourage them to turn to their clergyman or a trusted friend.

How Grandparents Can Help

After the first turmoil of facing the child's disorder has passed, some parents find that the child's grandparents are able to begin offering considerable emotional support. In other families, it is necessary for parents to recognize the limits of what grandparents can provide and to seek the understanding and comfort they need from their friends, brothers and sisters, from parents of other children with the same disorder, or from professional persons. Even in these families, however, the grandparents can often respond if parents suggest tangible ways of helping, perhaps some of the following:

1. Transporting or accompanying the child and parent to the doctor (especially helpful if the parent cannot drive, feels apprehensive about driving, or if the child is feeling sick, irritable or needs physical help).

2. Visiting the ill child during hospitalization.

3. Helping with the household routine (cleaning, cooking, marketing, repairs, errands).

4. Offering special attention and activities to brothers and sisters, who may be feeling left out.

5. Baby-sitting so that parents can have some opportunities to experience companionship as husband and wife.

Grandparents and Your Child

A child's illness or disability often alters the way his grandparents (aunts and uncles, too) behave around him and toward him. His condition may become the center of attention during every family gathering; conversation about his condition may be carried on over and around him, sometimes as though he weren't even there. On the other hand, his illness may never be mentioned at all; it may be treated as though it were a shameful secret.

Grandparents may begin to shower the child with extra attention, gifts, and special treats, and to be indulgent about any form of behavior he chooses to display. They may, on the other hand, begin to avoid him and seem quite fearful of being alone with him (and thus responsible for his well-being).

In each such instance, the grandparents are responding to the disorder more than to the child (as a young man with Cooley's anemia remarked bitterly, "I was treated like a disease, not a human being"). The child must depend on his parents to take a stand, to assert his identity as a worthwhile individual. He is not, after all, merely a hemophiliac, a leukemic, a nephrotic, a fibrocystic. He is a boy or a girl who happens to have hemophilia or leukemia or nephrosis or cystic fibrosis.

It is difficult for many parents to ask — clearly and firmly — their own parents to alter their behavior toward a grandchild. If you find yourself unable to do this, there are three available alternatives. You may simply allow the undesirable situation to continue, although this will not be helpful for your child and will probably produce smouldering resentment in you. You may avoid the grandparents, although this will probably arouse some guilt and sadness in you, and perhaps a sense of loss in your child. You may, finally, seek professional counseling to develop more effective family relationships. The third choice is the only one likely to benefit your parents, you, and your child.

3

Coping with Impaired Health
in the Infant and Toddler

Baby's Needs and Your Grief

Babies need food and shelter. They need also to be touched and cuddled and carried, spoken to and smiled at and played with. Babies need consistent care from one or two special people whom they can learn to know, to trust, and to love. Although father may help significantly, it is usually mother who is expected to provide the basic nurturance. This may be difficult indeed for mothers of babies with potentially serious health impairments.

Sometimes such mothers, grieving deeply, feel weighed down by sadness and fatigue. Lacking in energy or interest, they may find it a monumental task to respond to the baby's simplest need. Caring for him may seem an overwhelming effort.

Some mothers consciously fear emotional bonds: "I don't dare let myself get too attached to my baby. If something were to happen to him, I wouldn't be able to bear it." Such mothers try to avoid allowing the baby to arouse their tender feelings. They may try to give essential care without becoming deeply involved. They may limit contact with him as much as possible. Alternately, because they feel troubled by their wish to avoid contact, they may require themselves to be almost constantly at his side, constantly vigilant.

Some mothers feel discouraged because there is so little satisfaction in caring for their ill baby. Healthy babies pat and snuggle, gurgle and coo, smile and laugh, and thus charm their parents into responding. Their gain and growth and rapid development afford mother a sense of accomplishment that readily offsets the moments when child care is tiring and tiresome. She sees the evidence of a job well done, and her self-respect and self-confidence are enhanced. In contrast, the ill baby may be irritable, listless, puny, pale; he may grow and gain slowly. Abnormalities in his appearance or in his bodily products (stools and mucus, for example) may be distasteful to his mother. Outsiders, rather than complimenting her on her attractive offspring, may react to unusual aspects of his appearance or to outward symptoms, such as a cough. Their curious glances may seem to convey, "What have you done to your child?" Such a baby's mother is deprived of much pleasure in his care.

Indeed, there may be many moments when his care is burdensome and when she, understandably, resents this burden.

It is difficult indeed for the mother weighed down by her grief, the mother who fears becoming attached to her ill baby, the mother who is deprived of satisfaction from infant care, to touch and cuddle and carry, speak to and smile at, and play with the ill infant. This difficulty may influence both. The infant may want for the care that can help him thrive physically, emotionally, and intellectually. His mother, probably sensing that she is not fully meeting his needs, may reproach herself for her "failure," and her emotional burden will thus be increased.

How may such an impasse be resolved? First, such a mother — perhaps you are one — must find the courage to acknowledge, "Just now, I'm not able to care for my baby as I wish I could. I need help."

Emotional Support. Help with your feelings of sadness, anxiety, resentment, and guilt can be found (Chapters 1 and 8). Sharing, understanding, and coming to accept your feelings about your ill baby can lighten your emotional burden; it can make energy available to meet his needs; it can free you to make realistic judgments about what you feel able — and unable — to do for him.

Child Care Assistance. Help with child care may also be needed, at least temporarily. If a willing neighbor, friend, or relative is not available on a regular basis, money spent on a baby-sitter can be an essential investment (as important as the haircut, shoes, or dental care you probably would not hesitate to spend money on — and maybe more so). A skillful baby-sitter can give you necessary periods of relief from the child care which, at the moment, is not satisfying for you; he or she can also help to meet the baby's need for the attention, cuddling, and gentle stimulation which you may be feeling emotionally unable to provide. Should you find yourself reluctant to arrange or accept such help, or unable to justify the expense, it would be wise to explore your feelings of hesitation. Might you not be trying to atone for feelings of guilt about your baby's illness by bearing a staggering burden? Such attempts rarely benefit mothers, babies, or other family members.

Special Strategies of Child Care. There are various ways to help compensate for what you might feel unable to provide. A pediatrician, child psychologist, nursery school teacher, or hospital play therapist can be helpful in guiding you. For example, if you find yourself unable to talk or sing to your baby, you might play records for him. If you shrink from cuddling your baby, you might encourage your baby-sitter to caress him, and perhaps to massage his limbs gently. You might supply your baby with a few very soft, stuffed animals, and perhaps place a small cushion of smooth, silky fabric next to his skin. You might borrow a cradle for him to sleep in instead of a bassinet so that he can be soothed by the motion it provides.

The Feeding Experience

Giving food is the nucleus of mothering. It is the earliest way a mother can show tenderness and give satisfaction to her baby. It is the earliest way he can receive it. When a baby accepts nourishment from her and thrives, the mother's sense of accomplishment and worth is enhanced. If baby refuses her nourishment, or if he fails to thrive in spite of it, his mother's confidence may be shaken. She may feel that she is somehow failing her baby or that he is rejecting her care. Her uneasiness and urgency about feeding are sensed by the baby; he may, in fact, learn to refuse food as a way of asserting his self-hood. He may learn that refusals generate interesting attention and excitement. Even healthy babies and their parents express complicated attitudes about themselves and each other through the feeding situation. The presence of illness can increase the intensity and complexity of such feelings.

Encouraging Food Intake

Some illnesses cause babies to absorb and utilize their food ineffectively; their growth may be poor, they may appear thin and frail. Some illnesses result in poor appetite and little interest in food. In some illnesses it is medically urgent that a high level of intake be maintained. In all such instances, parents have a most realistic basis for concern.

In other illnesses, babies may remain well nourished but the concern of their parents may nevertheless be just as intense. Mothers (and fathers) tend to think of a baby with a health problem as being vulnerable, endangered. Nourishing him extra well — "building him up" — may seem like a kind of insurance that will safeguard him. Furthermore, although there are many aspects of an illness that parents cannot change, feeding offers one channel through which they can actively strive to help their baby. If they feel somehow responsible for the disorder, the need to help in this way may be especially strong. Mothers of healthy babies feel hurt if the baby rejects their love-offering of food. A mother who already feels at fault because her baby is ill may find such a rejection unbearable.

Although they are repeatedly advised, "Act casual," "Don't urge," such mothers are likely to approach feeding with feelings of urgency and tension that they cannot just "switch off," and which, unfortunately, babies quickly sense. Some babies respond to such tension by doing just exactly what their mothers fear — refusing food more and more.

If you are worried about feeding your baby, it can be helpful to analyze your approach to feeding. For example, as mealtime approaches, do you find yourself feeling tense, grim, determined, and fearful about the outcome? Can you spot ways in which your sense of urgency influences your feeding techniques? For example, do you find yourself rapidly thrusting the bottle or spoon into baby's mouth, or do you allow him to set the pace by signaling when he is ready (by turning his head toward the food and opening his mouth)? Do you hold bottle, cup, or spoon for him although he is able to do so himself? Do you respect his signals that he has had enough — clamping his lips shut, turning his head away, or shoving away the spoon, or do you insist on "just one more"?

Unfortunately, through such techniques you are likely to defeat your own purpose. The more strongly you insist, the more strongly your baby may resist. A negative attitude is likely to be aroused that can diminish his pleasure in eating and further reduce his appetite. There are no "TENSION-OFF" buttons for worried mothers to press. There are, however, a few approaches that can be helpful.

Clarifying the Reality. Although you doubtless have your own, private ideas about what foods are good for your baby, it is important to learn from his doctor whether there are special foods your baby requires. It is important also to learn whether food should be offered at set intervals of time and in particular amounts, or whether you can be flexible in designing a feeding "program." A professional dietitian can usually offer helpful suggestions about methods of preparing or presenting food so that it will be enticing to infants and young children; for example, tiny portions, small utensils, bright colors, crispy textures, are all appealing.

Respecting the Baby's Individuality. Your infant is likely to have his own, individual feeding rhythm. He may do best on frequent small feedings; he may accept food more eagerly at certain times of day. He may be a rapid gulper or a slow, dainty taster. He may need frequent pauses during a feeding, or he may take in the whole feeding nonstop. He may have definite preferences for one food over another of comparable nutritional value. If you try to attune yourself to these individual characteristics, feeding may be accomplished more smoothly.

Encouraging Mastery. As skill in grasping increases and coordination between hand and mouth improves, babies enjoy opportunities to participate in the feeding. Providing your infant or toddler with a tiny spoon to work with, a nonspill infant cup, a variety of finger foods, can increase his satisfaction in the mealtime experience.

Setting the Stage.   A mealtime that is as relaxed and pleasant as possible for you and your baby is likely to be the most successful one. It is worthwhile observing what conditions help you both to feel relaxed. For example, in which room does feeding seem to be most enjoyable? Does background music help? Does your baby show more interest in meals when he is alone with you — or when in the midst of family activity? Is it better if you sit with him through the whole meal or occasionally turn away to something else in the room? If you cannot avoid feeling tense under any circumstances, it might be wise to ask another family member to feed your baby, at least some of the time. A baby's interest in food is often enhanced if it is offered by a calm but responsive adult (or teenager) who can turn mealtime into a pleasant, social experience.

Restricting Food

In some disorders, the doctor may advise limitation of certain foods. Fortunately, it is rare that the baby's total diet must be restricted so much that he becomes hungry. More usually, there are only certain categories of food that should be limited; for example, salty foods for an infant with kidney disease, fatty foods for an infant with cystic fibrosis, sweets for a diabetic infant.

Babies don't yet understand that confections or snack foods are considered especially desirable; therefore they have no basis for feeling deprived if such foods are restricted. However, their parents may feel very uncomfortable about a limited diet. Not only is giving food at the very core of mothering, but in many families treat foods are used to symbolize love and approval. Withholding special foods may seem to parents like withholding love; parents who must do this sometimes feel mean.

Families deal with such food restrictions in different ways. In some households, the whole family is deprived of the forbidden food in order to avoid saying no to the baby. The foods are not offered at mealtime and, in fact, may never be brought into the household (unless a family member manages a successful smuggling operation). The M. family, whose toddler, Linda, was on a strict diet to keep her PKU (phenylketonuria) under control, went to great lengths to avoid allowing Linda to see them eating. They feared that she would beg for the foods they were eating, and they might find it unbearable to say no. Mrs. M. restricted herself to coffee for breakfast, and her husband ate en route to his office. She had lunch while Linda was napping, and dinner was postponed until ten o'clock, after Linda was in bed.

Such maneuvers are rarely constructive. First, they create an artificial situation for the child, who sooner or later must be exposed to food experiences outside the immediate family and should be learning at home to accept the limitations of his diet. Second, the deprivation usually begins to arouse the family's resentment. It is difficult to avoid becoming angry at the baby whose condition is the cause of this deprivation. Thus, the family's burden of troubled feelings is increased.

In some households, only the ill baby is deprived; the restricted foods are served to others. However, when the baby joins the family at mealtime, he shows a natural interest in what others are eating; he is likely to point at or reach for the foods he is not allowed. It can be most distressing for his parents to be repeatedly saying, "No, no," and perhaps to be having mealtime disrupted by baby's protests and tears. A mother who already feels guilty about the baby's disorder may become especially upset.

When either of these ways of managing a diet becomes too disturbing, the diet is apt to be neglected. The troubled mother is likely to become lax about restrictions, perhaps trying to convince herself that the baby's health is not suffering. Indeed, her efforts may already have been undermined by well-meaning relatives or friends, who urge, "Oh, let him have a little of that. Surely a taste couldn't harm him." Grandparents who find it difficult to accept the baby's disorder are especially prone to sabotage of this sort.

The most effective solution is one that takes into account the needs of all family members. Such a solution is usually a compromise. If french fries are served to the family only occasionally, a mother may comfortably say no to her baby, perhaps providing an interesting finger food as substitute. (After all, even healthy babies are not permitted all the food served to adults.) The other children may feel quite cheerful about having chocolate pudding only rarely at the family dinner if they can enjoy a pudding in their own lunchboxes or on a picnic. Parents who feel comfortable about management of the diet find it easier to be firm with relatives who suggest "just a taste" of forbidden foods.

Bodily Movement and Activity

Babies move because they must. There is an inborn need for movement, a motor drive. Satisfaction of this urge provides pleasure; interference with it may produce anger and anxiety. In addition, however, movement plays a complex and important role in the infant's and toddler's total development. If movement is restricted because of a medical disorder, the infant may be affected in significant ways.

The Importance of Movement

Movement releases tension and expresses emotion. The infant signals that he is hungry or chilly or startled by crying, but he also releases his misery by "bicycling" his legs, flailing his arms, arching his back. The toddler reacts to frustration by pushing, hitting, kicking, or biting. Pleasure is expressed through movement as well. The infant's body seems to go into a paroxysm of excitement at the sight of his bottle; the toddler jumps with joy when he is delighted.

Movement contributes to the growing sense of separateness and individuality that is one of the building blocks of personality development. The young infant at first lacks any sense of "I am me." The movement of his body in space and against the surfaces of his physical environment and the sensations such movement produces within him help the baby to learn how his body works; they help him to develop awareness of the boundaries of his body and to recognize that he is distinct from his environment. Movement toward and away from his mother (and others who care for him) helps him to realize that he and his mother are separate beings and enables him gradually to assert his growing sense of independence.

Movement provides social experience. The baby's movements arouse responses in those around him. The tiny baby turns his head toward the nipple, and mother feels satisfied; during feeding, he may touch, pull, fondle mother's body, and she feels tenderness or amusement, sometimes irritation. As mother approaches, the infant may lift his arms as though asking to be picked up. When held, the infant may clutch his mother's nose, grab her eyeglasses, pull her hair, stroke her cheek. All such movements cause mother, and others, to respond by smiling, talking, moving toward him; person-to-person contacts take place.

Movement promotes learning. From the moment he is first able to reach toward an object and grasp it, the infant moves his body in order to explore his world and, increasingly, to understand and influence it. He learns about softness and hardness, roughness and smoothness, coolness and warmth by grasping, stroking, twisting, crumpling, patting, licking, sucking, biting. He learns about size and weight and shape by pushing, pulling, lifting, and arranging. The toddler learns about direction and space by running, climbing, falling, chasing, dropping, and throwing. As his muscular skills develop, so may develop his sense of mastery. No longer feeling totally helpless, at the mercy of the world around him, he senses his growing capacity to manipulate and control at least small parts of it. This sense of mastery may have a very special value for the infant or toddler with impaired health, since at times his helplessness and dependence on others may be much greater than that of the healthy baby.

Interference with movement may affect the infant or toddler in several important ways. It may deprive him of a major source of pleasure. It may lead to the storing up of tension and excitement. It may impede his developing sense of individuality. It may reduce opportunities for social experience. It may interfere with learning. It may, in fact, give him the appearance of being mentally slow, even if his capacity for development and learning is entirely normal.

Interference with movement may result from the disorder itself. The infant may at times be listless and droopy. Certain illnesses may cause him to become short of breath or tired sooner than a healthy infant, and to stop his activity for a rest period more often.

Interference with movement may result from his parent's concern. Activity, bodily movement, is, in fact, one of the major worries of parents of ill children. Parents of children with hemophilia or osteogenesis imperfecta fear, with reason, that activity may result in a hemorrhage or a fracture. Parents of children with heart or lung or kidney or blood disease fear, understandably, that if they excite their babies or allow them to overdo, the infant's life may be endangered. Such parents may feel truly relaxed only when their babies are asleep or contentedly confined to crib or playpen.

An effective and realistic program of activity for a baby with impaired health must take into account the importance of movement for his social, emotional, and mental development, the limitations of activity caused by his disorder, and his parents' need to feel that he is safe. Several measures can be helpful in achieving these goals.

Helpful Measures

Collaborating with Professionals.   Decisions about your infant's activity need to be made in partnership with his doctor. Only he can inform you whether bodily movement offers any danger to your baby. He may, indeed, be able to offer considerable reassurance. For example, he knows that many babies with heart disease instinctively limit their activity; they sense when rest is needed and become quiet. Infants with lung disease may cough when they are active. Although parents may fear that this is harmful, the doctor may point out that the coughing helps to clear out secretions. Infants with hemophilia tend to have some unexplained bleeding episodes; they may also withstand some knocks and bumps without any bleeding. Your baby's doctor can share with you the responsibility for developing an activity program, and may also refer you to an experienced occupational therapist, physiotherapist, or rehabilitation counselor for advice. Some aspects of your baby's activity that you may find it helpful to talk over with such consultants are discussed below.

Offering Realistic Protection. If the baby is especially prone to bodily injury, it could be helpful to pad his crib and playpen heavily and to make at least one room in your house as accident proof as possible (perhaps with a thick, well-anchored rug, stable chairs, and tables with rounded corners). It would be wise to ask the doctor whether protective clothing — a "crash helmet," extra padding for arms and legs — would enable your baby to enjoy free movement more safely.

Offering Passive Movement. If your baby is inactive, or if his spontaneous movement is restricted, he can still experience beneficial motion if he is rocked, carried about securely enclosed in a papoose-type carrier, or allowed to spend some time in a well-constructed doorway swing. He may also benefit from gentle massage and from having his limbs moved in passive exercise. Should you feel tense and fearful about handling him in such ways, a calm relative or baby-sitter might be taught to give such care.

Bringing Baby onto the Scene. It is easy to allow a listless, inactive infant or toddler to spend much of his day in solitude, particularly if he accepts this without protest. Because he does not vigorously seek human contact, such a baby may particularly need to spend periods in whatever part of the home there is family activity. Even as a quiet observer in his infant seat or playpen, he will benefit from watching and hearing his family in action. He will profit further because those around are likely to smile at him, talk to him, touch him, and play with him just because he is there.

Indeed, communication by talking or singing can be most helpful. Long before he understands the ideas represented by words, the baby can sense the emotion conveyed in his parent's voice. Therefore, in talking to the baby, the adult is making a significant person-to-person contact, one that invites response from the baby. Even infants whose energy is at a low ebb because of illness usually respond. Their fretfulness may quiet; they may smile; they may vocalize in return. Voice games — cooing, babbling, imitating each other's sounds or words — form an important mode of play between adult and baby. Babies who are inactive physically often have sufficient energy for such communications.

Encouraging Play.   An active infant or toddler strives to use his whole environment as his playroom and every object in it as his toy. To have ample opportunity for learning about his world, an inactive or restricted baby needs to have playthings brought to him. He needs objects of various textures, sizes, and shapes; objects he can pat and squeeze, open and close, put together and take apart, fill and empty, sit on or throw. For an older infant, objects he has seen his mother use (a coffee pot, measuring spoons, an empty milk carton with some clothespins) have special appeal.

Too many playthings, offered or dropped into his playpen at once, may be confusing, even overwhelming, and stifle his natural interest. It is wiser to present two or three items at a time. Even then, an inactive infant may need to have his interest aroused. He may need an adult or older child to act as a playmate for a while, encouraging him to investigate his playthings (perhaps by showing him what can be done with them), and then continuing to express interest and approval from time to time. The baby learns from his play, and it can later serve a most important function in helping him endure his medical experiences.

Evaluating Development.   Some infants with extended illness show slow progress in motor development. They are later than most babies in accomplishing certain tasks of development involving bodily movement, posture and coordination (for example, sitting unsupported, standing alone, walking). Furthermore, experiences related to illness, such as hospitalization, may delay speech development or the baby's capacity to play and to respond to other people. As a result, their parents (and sometimes their doctors as well) fear that the baby is retarded or mentally slow.

Not only is this an additional source of anguish for the parents but babies viewed as retarded are also often handled differently from those viewed as normal or bright. If such a question arises, it is important to have your baby's development carefully evaluated. Only certain doctors — pediatricians who have specialized in the study of child development — are fully qualified to do this. A competent evaluation can also be carried out by a child psychologist experienced in examining infants. In most instances, such a specialist will be able to reassure you that your baby's capacity for intellectual development and learning is entirely normal.

Assertiveness and Home Treatment

Long before he can be aware that he and his mother are separate beings, the infant is capable of actions that seem to oppose her wishes and assert his own. At first, he may only be able to turn his head away from the nipple or spoon and clamp his lips tightly shut. He soon becomes able to push away the bottle or mother's hand as well. When first he can sit up unaided, he can protest only with tears, twisting, and turning, the indignity of being thrust down on his back — for bodily care such as a diaper change; later, he can crawl away from mother and, as a toddler, he can run (perhaps looking back in anticipation of an exciting chase). Thus, as his sense of his own individuality and his need to assert his independence develop, so do the bodily skills to oppose mother in a widening variety of ways.

Often reaching a peak around 18 months, the baby's negativism may remain at a very high level for a year or more. Whether or not he enjoys saying no — and in spite of his deep need for loving approval — the toddler often *has* to say no. The more grimly determined you become that he should do something, the more insistent he may become that he won't.

Many babies with an extended illness require a regimen of home treatment that may include medications given by mouth or by injection, inhalation therapy, and bodily manipulations, such as physiotherapy and postural drainage. Even though parents know that home treatment offers a constructive way of helping their sick child, they may, for various reasons, feel tense and grim about it. Treatment may interrupt family activities and take time away from other important tasks. Parents may worry that they will not carry out the treatment correctly and effectively. Treatment is a recurrent and insistent reminder that baby has an illness even if he appears quite healthy. Doing the treatment may arouse in parents an upsurge of their grief and of resentment because they and their baby are so burdened. If treatment is uncomfortable, or frankly painful for the child, parents feel distressed and perhaps also guilty at causing the pain.

A baby's need to oppose his parents' wishes and to assert his own may combine with his parents' distress to turn treatment into a battle scene. The mother's tension may lead her to respond to the infant's first protest with grim insistence, which provokes him to stronger refusal, which makes her angry (because she is frightened she won't succeed), which impels him to struggle furiously — and so a vicious circle is set in motion. At such times, parents may feel desperate enough to try to subdue the infant's protests with slaps and spanks. Although an occasional slap is scarcely a catastrophe, if stormy scenes occur frequently, the infant is likely to experience treatment as a punishment which he will learn to dread. The parent, in turn, may find the experience so upsetting that she begins to avoid treatment, perhaps putting it off or forgetting to carry it out.

There are techniques that can help to interrupt such a vicious cycle or, better yet, to prevent it from developing.*

Helpful Measures

Examining Your Own Feelings.   It is natural to have moments of feeling apprehensive or resentful or regretful about your baby's treatment. It is understandable to feel frightened or to lose your temper occasionally if he fights against treatment. Facing your feelings and attitudes about the treatment as honestly as possible enables you to plan a realistic program, one that takes into account your needs as well as your baby's. A regimen that fails to do this rarely works for very long.

Enhancing Self-confidence.   Infants are quick to sense tension in an adult giving care. If you have any questions or feelings of uncertainty about treatment techniques, it is wise to ask for additional demonstrations by a professional therapist and for supervision of your method of giving treatment at home. Even parents experienced in giving home treatment feel reassured by an occasional review of the procedures with the doctor, a public health nurse, a physiotherapist, or an inhalation therapist. Usually, however, the parent must take the responsibility for requesting the review.

Planning the Treatment Timetable Thoughtfully.   The doctor will be able to tell you how frequently treatments should be given, whether they should be given before or after meals, whether it is necessary to continue them through the night. He can also let you know whether it is permissible to be somewhat flexible, so that your treatment timetable can take into account the pattern of your baby's activity, the needs of other family members, and your own moods. For example, it would be inviting protest if you were to snatch your infant away for treatment while he is involved in a delightful game of peek a boo with the child from next door; it is tactful to give treatment when your infant is in transition between activities rather than in the midst of one. If there is a certain period

*Some important issues concerning treatment are discussed in Chapter 8.

every day when he tends to have a cranky spell (or when you are apt to feel tired and irritable), it would be wise to avoid giving treatment at such a time if possible. If the baby usually responds to treatment with excitement and protest, it would be preferable not to carry it out just at bedtime. If the treatment time cannot be changed, perhaps bedtime should be postponed long enough to allow for a soothing, quiet recovery period. Similarly, it would be unfortunate to begin your infant's or toddler's treatment just as your first grader is dismounting from the school bus and running in to tell you about his day.

Some flexibility is helpful, but too much may be burdensome if the treatment seems to be hanging over your head much of the time. For example, if you think about a 15-minute treatment for an hour before you actually do it, the treatment will have taken up 75 minutes of your mental life. Many parents find it effective to build treatment into the day, much as they build in dressing, washing, or brushing teeth. Treatment thus takes on the character of habit, and the amount of conscious decision making involved is reduced.

Setting the Stage.   Treatment may be simplified if preparations are made before you bring the baby on the scene. If the treatment procedure is a brief one, you may need only to gather and prepare the equipment (such as medicine, spoon, dropper, sterile hypodermic, or alcohol swab) in advance. In the case of more prolonged and complex treatment, such as inhalation therapy and postural drainage, it is helpful to set the stage so that you can feel as relaxed as possible. Parents find that doing the treatment in a bright, cheerful room or turning on some lighthearted music may lift their spirits. A well-chosen television program (nothing grim or sad) can help a parent relax, and even an infant can become interested in the changing images and sounds. It may help a toddler endure the treatment if he is told or read a simple story or if a brother or sister stays within his field of vision. It may help if he is given something to hold that he enjoys feeling and manipulating.

Encouraging an Active Role.   Your infant has an increasing need to assert his wishes and play an active role in the events of his life. Finding appropriate ways for these needs to be met in home treatment is a challenge to your ingenuity. Each time an infant reaches a new level of bodily mastery (sitting up alone, pulling to stand, taking the first steps), he seems to feel outraged when he is deprived of his new accomplishment by having his body placed in a more helpless and "babyish" position — being made to lie down, for example. It protects his sense of dignity and minimizes his need to protest if, as far as is reasonable, he is allowed to sit or stand while bodily manipulations are being carried out.

A toddler can be offered some choices in the treatment situation, but it is essential that you offer a choice only when you are willing to accept his decision. Asking, "Shall we take the medicine now?" is inappropriate since your toddler will surely say "no"; asking, "Would you like grape juice or orange juice after your medicine?" allows for acceptable choosing.

The toddler can also be encouraged to imitate the giving of treatment in his play with a doll or stuffed animal. Through such play, in which he is the active doer rather than the passive and helpless receiver, young children express and master some of the fear and anger treatment can arouse. Although preschool children are able to use this channel more effectively than toddlers, the toddler can be encouraged to begin developing this capacity. For example, before the nebulizer mask is placed over his face for inhalation therapy, you might suggest that your toddler cover a stuffed animal's snout and give it a treatment. After he has received an injection in his own thigh, your toddler may vent his indignation by repeatedly giving shots to any available victims. Of course, only a toy hypodermic or a stuffed animal patient should be used. Family pets, as well as brothers and sisters, may need to be protected.

Choosing the Home Therapist.   Some parents, at some times, find it impossible to carry out home treatment with a reasonable degree of confidence, skill, and relaxation. Difficult as it is to admit to yourself (let alone to the doctor), "I just can't do it," such an admission may be the most effective way to help your baby at that time. It frees you to stop avoiding or postponing treatment, to accept your own distress, and to consider who is available to share the responsibility for a while. Your spouse, another relative, a close friend or neighbor who has often said, "Let me know how I can help," might be considered. Your child's doctor or the public health nurse in your community may be able to help you locate and train someone to do home treatment. A voluntary health agency may be able to put you in touch with other parents of similarly afflicted children who are interested in sharing responsibility for home treatment.

Impulse Control

The Need for Control

As he grows and develops, the baby becomes able to express all of his impulses — aggressive and loving, self-assertive and oppositional, exploratory and acquisitive — in a widening variety of direct actions. He grabs, pushes, throws, drops, climbs, jumps, runs toward and away, according to his whims. If thwarted, he not only cries but also may hit, kick, bite, hurl his body around, and bang his head.

His capacity to think about his actions, or to recall the past and anticipate the future, is only gradually beginning to develop as he becomes a toddler. It is hard for him to wait for satisfaction of his wants, and most difficult to understand the possible results of what he does. Therefore, he depends on those who care for him to help him regulate his behavior. He seems to feel reassured when he is protected from hurting himself or others or from destroying property.

In time, from a need for love and approval as well as a wish to behave as his parents do, he will begin to develop his own inner controls. These controls will at first be uncertain. The older toddler may try to quell his impulses by behaving in a strikingly opposite way. For example, struggling against the impulse to mess, he may become fastidiously clean, objecting strenuously to the tiniest speck on his hand or in his food. He may deal with resentment against a new baby by being excessively, unbelievably loving. He may also welcome routines and develop elaborate ceremonies at special times such as bedtime to help him in his task of self-regulation. For many years, however, the guidance and support of adults will be urgently needed.

It is particularly helpful if regulation and discipline are offered in a way that safeguards the baby's budding sense of dignity and that also allows him some freedom to explore his world and test his skills. Too many angry confrontations in which the baby is usually the loser are hard on his precarious self-esteem, and can turn the household into a battleground. Too many no's can interfere with his drive to learn. An understanding mother (or father) will baby proof some areas of the home by removing breakable objects, covering electrical outlets, securing tippy furniture, and locking away the poisons. An understanding mother will intervene early and quickly when trouble is beginning to develop, rather than waiting until a showdown is needed. An understanding mother will offer a diversion or an acceptable substitute when it is necessary to say no. An understanding mother will offer acceptable outlets in play for the baby's impulses to smear, mess, pound, squeeze, twist, throw.

To be sure, the most understanding mother becomes tired, harassed, irritable, and may be provoked to an angry outburst against the toddler. Fortunately, most human relationships can absorb some anger. The baby will, however, need comfort and reassurance as soon as his mother (or father) feels genuinely able to offer it. If the mother has a sense of self-respect and a confident awareness of her loving feelings toward the baby, it is not difficult to say, "Yes, I did get angry because you tipped over the lamp, but we all make mistakes, and I do still love you."

Problems in Setting Limits

Parents of children with impaired health may have particular difficulty in helping their babies learn to regulate and control their impulses. There are several possible reasons for such difficulty. Parents may fear that upsetting or angering their baby by interfering with his behavior or frustrating his wishes might be physically harmful. They fear that the anger might bring on an acute episode of the illness, such as a convulsion, an asthmatic attack, or that it might overstrain a damaged heart. Such fears are understandable when a baby's physical state is precarious. However — and this should certainly be discussed with your baby's doctor — it is likely that your baby's health will be taxed more severely if there is a continuous buildup of tension between a demanding little tyrant and his resentful family.

A mother who is unable to dispel her feelings of responsibility and guilt concerning the baby's disorder may have a need to make it up to the baby by indulging all his wishes and tolerating any behavior. If the baby in such a case becomes a tyrant — and he most surely will — his disagreeable behavior amply punishes his parent, and the guilt may be somewhat relieved.

A baby's extended illness, which is realistically a frustration and a burden, almost inevitably produces some feelings of resentment and anger in his parents. Many a parent feels ashamed of this resentment, and tries to bottle it up and conceal it. Because a confrontation with a demanding, disobedient, or aggressive infant may cause the bottle to blow out its cork, and the hidden anger to flow out, such a parent may make every effort to avoid the confrontations that threaten to release the anger.

Some parents who feel burdened and resentful live in a state of intense inner tension. An explosive scene may be necessary to allow them to vent their anger and temporarily clear the air. Without being aware of this need, they find themselves permitting the infant to behave more and more disagreeably until, finally, a monumental outburst of anger seems justified.

Some parents, curiously, need to express their own inner anger and protest through their child's behavior. Unable to voice their resentment about the misfortune of his illness, it is as though they silently say, "Good for you! Go to it!" each time the infant is aggressive or destructive.

Parents who have difficulty in guiding and regulating their infant's behavior are usually unaware of the underlying reasons. If such a difficulty is persistent, it can greatly benefit parent and child to explore the problem through professional counseling, in order to develop more effective ways of managing the parent's feelings and the infant's behavior. Although very strict control may offer constant frustration and interfere with the infant's and toddler's learning about himself and his world, continuous indulgence or confusingly inconsistent regulation encourages him to become a discontented tyrant. At the mercy of his strong urges and drives, he will feel anxious. Imperiously demanding, perhaps destructive, he will arouse resentment and anger in those around him that he will readily sense and that will intensify his anxiety and his misery. It will be very hard indeed for his parents to find any enjoyment in his company or his care.

Hospitalization and the Separation Experience

Most babies with extended illness need periods of hospitalization for diagnosis or treatment. For several reasons, this can be a particularly difficult experience during infancy. First, the infant is usually feeling ill at the time of hospitalization. Second, his parents, who are already sad and worried about his disorder, are likely to feel frightened and agitated as well when hospitalization is needed. Even a very young infant senses their distress through their tone of voice, facial expression and the tension in their muscles as they touch and hold him. Third, the hospital is a strange environment with strange sights, sounds, and smells. There are strange people, unfamiliar cribs or beds. The food is prepared differently, nursing bottles may have a different feel. Fourth, the infant is subjected to examinations and manipulations of his body that may be frightening and uncomfortable. His movement may need to be restrained. Fifth, and most important of all, hospitalization probably involves separation from his mother. The infant cannot be prepared for any of these experiences, nor can he understand the reasons for them. He is unable to express his own feelings and ideas or to ask meaningful questions.

The Significance of Separation

During the first months of life, the infant shows increasing interest in and response to those who care for him. However, he cannot yet distinguish Mother (or the person who plays the mothering role) from "not-

Mother." Around the middle of his first year (between four and eight months in most babies), the infant begins to respond differently to the Mother and the not-Mothers, thus showing that he is beginning to distinguish between them. He may become quiet and tense, gaze at the not-Mother with a searching and worried look, and then begin to cry. He seems to sense that he needs a particular mother to keep him comfortable and safe.

His experience of Mother is limited to what she does for and with him. He has no way of knowing that she has an existence all her own, apart from himself. Therefore, when his mother is absent, it is as though she had stopped existing. Brief separation can be worrying if a need arises that his mother is not there to meet. Longer separation can arouse deep anxiety.

Somewhere between 18 and 24 months, the toddler begins to be able to keep an image of Mother in his mind when she is absent. He begins to understand that she exists even when he does not see or hear her. He begins to realize that separation is followed by reunion. However, he still has no realistic sense of time. When he needs his mother — for cuddling, for bodily comfort, to help him control his strong impulses — he cannot easily wait. Being told that she will be there in five minutes, or after lunch, does not reassure him much.

Responses to Hospitalization

During the first few months of life, before he has developed a specific attachment to his mother, the infant may tolerate hospitalization quite well if he is well nurtured — cuddled, rocked, talked to, and played with by interested adults, such as nurses, aides, and volunteers, when his mother cannot be with him. If there are some reactions to the differences in feeding, sleeping, and bathing routines, they tend to be mild and temporary.

During these early months, separation is likely to be more troubling to the infant's mother than it is to him. As the infant is gradually learning to recognize his mother as a special person, and is developing a loving attachment to her, so is the mother developing her own emotional bonds to her baby and confidence in her capacity to care for him. Hospitalization may interfere with the growth of these bonds. The mother may feel that her baby is becoming a stranger to her, and she may lose confidence in her mothering skills. If he seems to be in danger, she may fear allowing an emotional attachment to grow. She may, in fact, believe that if he cannot recover full health, it might be more merciful if he would die. Such thoughts are profoundly troubling and make the mother's relationship with her hospitalized infant a very uneasy one.

In contrast to the infant of up to three or four months of age, the older baby is likely to show marked changes in behavior during hospitalization. There may be temporary emotional withdrawal, with a loss of interest in the environment and a lack of responsiveness to the people in it. This is a common response to acute illness; it is as though the baby needs to direct all his attention toward his sick body and to conserve his energy for recovery. In past years, such behavior might have also reflected the despair of babies whose mothers were forbidden to visit because of rigid hospital rules.

There may be regression; that is, recent accomplishments in the infant's or toddler's development may be lost, with a return to earlier patterns of behavior. With his energy needed to deal with the stress of being in the hospital, a toddler may, for example, lose interest in feeding himself, return to wetting and soiling, increase his thumbsucking. The development of language may be halted.

There may be protest behavior, with crying, fretfulness, temper outbursts, extreme rebelliousness, and negativism. There may be changes in the infant's sleeping, eating, and bowel habits.

The reactions may be widely varied. The baby needs — in fact he has a right — to react to the strange environment and worrying experiences. But his reactions can be troubling to his parents. Already worried about his bodily illness, they now must also face puzzling and perhaps disagreeable changes in his behavior and personality. They not only must find effective ways of comforting and reassuring him but also must deal with the sadness and apprehension and annoyance and guilt that his reactions may arouse in them.

What Helps?

Visiting.   Since separation from mother is the most crucial stress for the hospitalized infant, there are few things that can help him tolerate the experience more effectively than his mother's presence. The infant can, in fact, endure a remarkable amount of bodily discomfort and manipulation without adverse effects if he has this support. In recognition of this fact, during the past 20 years, most U.S. hospitals have relaxed their visiting regulations on children's services. Many provide facilities for mothers to live in with their babies, or they allow unrestricted visiting.

Mothers may also be encouraged to help care for their babies, especially by feeding, bathing, changing, dressing, and playing with them. In this way, mothers can maintain or increase their confidence in their nurturing skills, and learn how to respond to any special needs related to the illness. And so, even when the patient is so young that he might willingly accept substitute mothering, regular and frequent visiting is beneficial.

Mothers may, however, feel emotionally torn about visiting. They wish to be with the ill baby, to comfort and reassure him, to observe his condition and progress directly. On the other hand, visiting or living in may be difficult and upsetting. Many infants and toddlers can fully release their misery only in their mother's comforting presence. Although an outburst of crying relieves the baby and helps him endure hospitalization, it may arouse unbearable sorrow and regret in his mother. She may long to avoid this heartbreak, telling herself, "I just upset him when I go. He's better off without me."

Furthermore, the baby's condition may make it difficult to comfort him in familiar ways. If he is under restraint for an intravenous infusion, for example, he may seem reproachful and bewildered if his mother fails to pick him up when he turns toward her. Unable to explain, she may feel so distressed that it is difficult to stay.

The mother may even feel a sense of uneasiness the moment she steps into the hospital. The sights and smells may stir frightening memories of a childhood illness of her own, or reawaken sadness about the loss of a beloved relative or friend. Her discomfort may be intensified because she lacks the familiar, organizing influence of her usual routine of daily work.

Although for these and other reasons visiting may be disturbing, many parents do find ways to relieve their discomfort. For example, it can be supportive if a friend or relative can accompany you to the hospital. This comforting presence can help you endure your child's misery and comfort him in turn. A social worker or hospital chaplain may be available as a compassionate listener with whom you can share your distress. A wise nurse or play therapist may be able to suggest different ways of interacting with your baby if you cannot pick him up and cuddle him. For example, perhaps you might hold his hand, stroke his head, make his teddy bear or snoopy dog do a funny dance. You might sing to him softly or recite nursery rhymes, using the familiar sound of your voice to soothe him.

Other ·Ways of Helping. Some parents, because of continuing emotional discomfort, needs of other family members, or transportation problems, are not able to live in with the ill baby nor to visit every day, even if hospital policy encourages it. And other parents are, unfortunately, subject to rigid and restrictive hospital visiting policies. But in either instance there is still much that can be done to help the baby endure hospitalization if parents collaborate with the staff in trying to meet his needs.

Although you must depend on the staff for medical information, they must depend on you for information about your baby's individuality: his nickname, his food preferences, his bowel and sleeping habits, his special way of being comforted or of comforting himself. It may be helpful to write this information down and ask that it be included in the chart with the nursing notes. Further, the staff may depend on you to supply whatever special comforter — teddy bear, security blanket, special pillow, pacifier — seems to help your infant feel safe.

It is not easy for an infant to transfer his fragile sense of trust from his mother to the hospital staff. The older infant and toddler may be able to do this to some extent if he senses that you have confidence in the staff. It is helpful to find out who your baby's particular nurses will be.* Sharing with them your observations and concerns about your baby, and sensing their interest in his welfare, can strengthen your own sense of trust. Should you find yourself feeling hostile, or competitive, or constantly critical of the staff — as parents sometimes are — it is most important to try to work out such feelings. A social worker may be able to help you do this effectively.

It is helpful to talk over your visiting plans with the staff, and to cooperate with them in selecting the best times for the visits you are able to make. The choice may be influenced by your baby's medical needs (you may wish not to come while the doctors are making their rounds) as well as his emotional needs (a toddler experiencing separation anxiety may need you most at bedtime). Knowing of your plans, the staff may arrange to give your baby special comfort through the distress of your departure.

Leave-taking can be painful for parents. When a toddler realizes that you are going away, he is likely to cry miserably. Some parents attempt to avoid this heartrending scene by slipping away without saying goodbye. They hope the toddler will fail to notice or react to their absence. Though the parent's wish to avoid distress is understandable, the baby's sense of trust is better preserved if he is made aware that you are leaving. As you go, he can be consoled by his nurse. There may, in

*Hospital staff are assigned to patients either by task assignment (in which one nurse carries out particular functions such as bathing or feeding, with many different patients) or case assignment (in which the nurse carries out many different functions with a very few patients who are identified as her patients). Hospitals sensitive to the emotional needs of patients tend to prefer the latter, since it affords personal and individualized care.

fact, be many periods during your absence — if your plans are known — when nursing staff, aides, or volunteers can be assigned to your baby for substitute mothering.

Aftermath

Your baby's hospitalization is likely to distress you. It may also afford relief, since his care in the hospital is the responsibility of skilled professionals. As the time for his discharge approaches, you may feel both glad and apprehensive, since this responsibility will be transferred back to you. It is wise to ask for instruction from such professionals as nurses, dietitians, physiotherapists, and inhalation therapists. They can demonstrate the special techniques of care your child will continue to need, and then supervise you as you begin to develop skill in carrying them out.

Most babies continue to react to hospitalization for several weeks after discharge. Your baby may be irritable and whiny, cling to you and cry when you go even into another room, become tearful at bedtime, or be wakeful during the night. He may protest ordinary care of his body in ways that puzzle you until you understand the connection to his hospital experience. (An infant who had received many injections in the thighs and buttocks during hospitalization reacted to diaper changes for many weeks afterwards. Each time his mother unpinned and opened a wet or soiled diaper, his entire body would become tense and rigid, and he would begin to wail.) Your baby may — especially if you were unable to visit often — be unresponsive to you for a while and seem to have lost interest in people as well as playthings.

Are such reactions harmful? Perhaps the greatest risk is that they may influence your relationship with your baby in a negative way. Should his clinging or irritability or fearfulness make you feel annoyed or guilty (many parents feel both), you may respond to him with more tension or irritability than usual. This, in turn, can increase his clinging and crying and fretfulness, which further intensifies your annoyance and guilt. A vicious cycle is set in motion.

Expecting that your baby will probably react to hospitalization (so that you can accept his reactions without alarm), realizing that such reactions are usually temporary, allowing yourself as much help as possible during this difficult time — all such preparation can help prevent the vicious cycle. Should your baby's reactions seem unexpectedly intense or persistent, or should you find yourself feeling particularly troubled by his behavior, it can be valuable to talk over the problem with your pediatrician, a public health nurse, or a social worker.

4

Coping with Impaired Health in Early Childhood

Family Relations: Tenderness and Rivalry

The Growth of Tenderness and Rivalry

A baby's feelings of love arise in response to the care he receives — care that relieves him of disagreeable sensations, such as hunger, chilliness, or soreness, and provides pleasant ones instead. Although father and parent substitutes may play a significant role, it is usually his mother who gives such care. Therefore, during his first three years it is usually his mother whom the infant or toddler loves most intensely, whom he depends on most strongly for safety and comfort, whom he tries hardest to imitate, and at whom, in moments of frustration, he feels most angry.

By early childhood, however, he is striving to free himself from his intense, physical dependency on his mother. He has become increasingly capable of providing some of his own bodily care: feeding himself, going to the bathroom, washing and dressing. He is increasingly determined to do so. One of the most frequent declarations of the three-year-old is, "I can do it all by my own self!" To the chagrin of his parents, he may even reject needed help with difficult problems like buttons and shoelaces. Furthermore, he is increasingly capable of tolerating some separation from his mother and of accepting care and supervision from others.

Along with increasing independence, the young child is striving to achieve some sense of identity as boy-to-become-man or girl-to-become-woman. The developmental pathways toward these goals differ somewhat for boys and girls. However, the emotional relationships within the family play a crucial part, especially the complex "family triangle," the relationship of special tenderness toward one parent and rivalry toward the other that strongly influences love relationships later in life.

For the little boy, the intense attachment to mother that developed in infancy continues into early childhood, but usually changes its character. No longer content to be the helpless and dependent receiver of his mother's care, the boy imagines himself in a more active and aggressive relationship to his mother — her provider, her protector. He may strive to become her beloved partner — as his father is — and may declare his intention of marrying her later on. He feels moments of jealousy about his father's special position, fleeting feelings of rivalry toward him, and fleeting wishes that his father would go away forever. He also has uneasy moments when he imagines that his father may become angry at his small rival and punish him in a disagreeable or frightening way.

This intense and tender attachment between mother and son can be a treasured experience for both (few women fail to enjoy being regarded as so beautiful, wonderful, and wise as they are by their uncritical young sons). It can be a poignant moment in his mother's life when the child announces, "I'm sorry, Mom, but I won't be able to marry you after all." Several influences, however, do contribute to the loosening of the attachment. Mother probably gives less intimate care, because her growing son needs it less and because other responsibilities, perhaps the care of a younger child, claim her. Uneasiness about his feelings of rivalry toward his father and anxiety about arousing his father's displeasure exert their effect on the child. Finally, his advancing intellectual development enables him to be more realistic; he becomes aware that it is not possible to become his mother's mate. Gradually, the little boy gives up his striving to replace his father, and accepts the more attainable aim of becoming a man like father and one day finding a mate of his own.

Striving to outgrow her helpless, dependent relationship to her mother, but still having loving feelings toward her, the little girl also may imagine herself in an active role as her mother's protector. However, she is likely to abandon this idea much more swiftly than the boy does. Her drive toward independence, perhaps reinforced by disappointment if her mother has turned her interest toward a new baby, usually results in a partial turning away from her mother. Her father, instead, becomes the object of her tender feelings and daydreams. Father is most likely to respond to her affection and her adoration with his own special tenderness, and thus the father-daughter relationship may have the special sweetness of the attachment between mother and son, and be as treasured.

The relationship between mother and daughter may become quite troubled and characterized by contradictions. The little girl's struggle for independence impels her to resist and defy and oppose her mother, although she still needs her mother's care, and, when she is sad, weary, or hurt, she longs for her mother's comfort. The little girl feels rivalry with her mother for her father's interest and love, and some jealousy at her mother's privileged position. On the other hand, as she practices her role of girl-to-become-woman in her play and her daydreams, she needs to imitate and identify with her mother, who is, after all, her most important model of womanhood. Therefore, the little girl's defiant and rivalrous feelings toward her mother cause her some worry. What if she were to make her mother very angry? Might her mother punish her or go away and leave her?

The little girl's sense of sexual identity may remain uncertain for some time. It is influenced (as is the boy's) by the attitudes of her family and the values of her parents' ethnic group. If the child senses that boys are valued more highly, she may strive to behave in boyish ways in order to win approval.

Furthermore, although she comes to realize that she cannot become her father's wife, her competitive feelings toward her mother may continue until adolescence, intensified at times by a fresh drive toward independence. Around six years of age, for example, many docile and charming little girls bewilder and anger their mothers by becoming defiant, rude, and obnoxious — "brats" — as they are faced with the serious reality of a full school day and struggle against their longing to stay in a warm, safe home.

For one parent, the period of the family triangle may be a delight and a time of special tenderness. For the other, it may be a troubled time. It is not easy to hear your child shriek, "I hate you — I wish you were dead!" or, "Go away, Daddy. Go back to your office. I don't want you. I want Mommy." At the end of the day, a weary mother may long for her husband's comforting hug and resent the little girl who dashes first into his arms. A father, in days of discouragement, may feel that his wife shows more enthusiasm for their son's feats in nursery school than his own in the practice of law.

Special difficulties face the single parent, whether unmarried, separated, divorced, or widowed. He or she may have to accept the full intensity of the child's affection, and bear the full brunt of his anger. He or she may also experience the pain of being blamed or resented for the absence of the other parent, for whom the child naturally has moments of longing.

The Influence of Illness

Both of the developmental tasks that have been described — loosening the dependent attachment to mother and developing a sense of sexual identity — are influenced by illness. Mothers of healthy children have mixed feelings about their child's increasing independence. It is a source both of pride ("He's so big and capable") and of a sense of loss ("He needs me less now"). Illness may make it even more difficult to give up responsibility for bodily care, both because the child appears frail, helpless, and vulnerable and because of his medical needs. For example, rather than encouraging independence in toiletting, the mother may have to collect urine specimens or inspect the child's bowel movements. Anxiety about the child's nutrition, or the need for a special diet, may cause the parent to continue feeding the child or supervising his eating habits longer and more closely than she would with a healthy child. Concern about such bodily changes as swelling or bruising may cause the parent to participate in bathing or dressing the child more constantly than otherwise. The parent may feel a need to sleep with the child at night to reassure herself that he's really all right. Home treatments, such as postural drainage, may require placing the child's body in passive and helpless positions, as though he were a baby.

Some young children may accept such care willingly, and seem to enjoy the helplessness and passivity. It can be enjoyable indeed to be the object of the mother's special interest and attention. A little girl may, therefore, be delayed in turning toward father as the special object of her tender feelings. A little boy may find it difficult to give up his intense, close attachment to his mother. If his mother becomes so absorbed in his care that she seems to have little interest in father, that can seem especially nice — until the boy begins to sense that his father doesn't enjoy it so much and is feeling some resentment toward his son. Then his pleasure will be tarnished by uneasiness. Furthermore, the child — whether boy or girl — is also deprived of the feeling of competence and self-mastery that grows with increasing independence and that is a foundation of the sense of personal worth.

Rather than being compliant, however, some children may need to resist the mother's care desperately and to engage in obstructive and defiant behavior that makes management of the disorder most difficult. Although some little girls, struggling to free themselves of too much dependence on their mothers, do show such behavior, it is probably more common among small boys. Beginning to understand that assertiveness, vigor, and independence are considered boyish, and that being gentle, helpless, timid and passively receiving care are considered girlish* (as well as babyish), the little boy may need to resist the dependent role desperately in order to protect his budding sense of manhood. His frantic resistance may make the management of his illness most difficult. It may include angry outbursts during which the parents may be blamed for the illness, accusations that are painful indeed for a troubled parent to hear.

*These traditional stereotypes are being modified in many sectors of U.S. society. Gentleness in a man is becoming accepted as appropriate, as is assertiveness in a woman.

Parents of healthy children experience momentary resentment, anger, and jealousy. Such feelings tend to occur more frequently and more intensely among parents of ill children. The illness may produce demanding, irritable behavior in the child. The illness is, realistically, a burden. One parent may become so absorbed in the child's care that the marriage is subject to strain.* For any such reasons, parents may find that their resentment and anger reach a peak that is quite worrying.

What Helps?

Studies of children with illnesses such as hemophilia and heart disease have shown that although they may outwardly accept a position of continuous helplessness and dependence, inwardly they are likely to feel anxious and resentful and — in time — have a low opinion of themselves. Naturally, when they feel acutely sick, children need and welcome intensive care. Much of the time, however, children with extended illnesses can take over considerable responsibility for their own bodily needs. If encouraged to do so, their feelings of self-confidence and of being worthwhile are greatly strengthened.

Some children are capable of considerable responsibility for their medical needs by four or five years of age. That is, they can cooperate actively with adults. They can learn to collect their own specimens, hold their own nebulizer,† pour juice to "wash down" their medicine, hold still for an injection. They can decide to rest when they feel tired or breathless, tell their mother if they have bruised themselves, learn to mark a chart showing how many glasses of water they have drunk. Your own child's doctor or a registered nurse can probably help you recognize many ways in which you and your child can share responsibility for his bodily care. It is important to ask directly for such advice.

Things can also be done to make the management of the family triangle as effective as possible. Foremost among these is to try to recognize ways in which the care of the child may be straining the marital relationship. Although small boys have daydreams about coming first in their mothers' affections — and little girls in their fathers' — they do, in fact, feel most secure when they sense that the relationship between their parents is secure. It is therefore of great importance that parents enjoy some periods alone as man and wife. It is also of great value to plan ways in which the child's father can have a meaningful role

---

*Some examples have been described in Chapter 2.

†Some ways in which the toddler can begin participating in his treatment have been suggested in Chapter 3. These are applicable to the young child as well.

in his care so that the father is not left out of an exclusive relationship between mother and child (as happened to Peter's father — described in Chapter 2).

Parents of an ill child, already sad, regretful, and perhaps guilty about the disorder, often have difficulty accepting even quite appropriate resentful feelings toward the child. Believing such feelings to be somehow wrong, they may strive desperately to conceal their resentment from others — and from themselves. Those who care about the family, relatives, friends, clergymen, doctors, and nurses, can serve them well by encouraging the parents to vent their resentment from time to time and by listening compassionately while they do so. An occasional gripe session can clear the air and make room for the feelings of love and concern that resentment can crowd out. Those who care about the family can encourage the parents to form a partnership in looking after the child. If both parents take some responsibility for the treatments and the trips to the doctor, it is less likely that one will become an outsider. Friends and relatives can also offer practical help — perhaps an evening of baby-sitting — so that the parents can renew their commitment to each other.

Fact and Fancy

Characteristics of Thought

"I wish I knew what he has on his mind," parents of children with extended illness often declare. A good deal is, in fact, known about the kinds of thoughts young children have about themselves and their experiences, and the kinds of theories they form about their bodies, birth, illness, and death.

The thoughts of young children are, first of all, highly personal, egocentric. Their ideas and theories are centered upon their own sensations, actions, emotions, and their everyday experiences with people and things. The young child is convinced of the rightness of his beliefs and has trouble understanding another viewpoint. However, his ideas may have little relationship to reality as his parents view it.

The thoughts of a young child reflect his confusion between his inner world and the outer world around him. He cannot clearly distinguish between his own thoughts, feelings, and mental images and the outside world of people, things, and events. For example, his fears take form in thoughts of evil shapes, shadows, monsters, and bogeymen; the child is at times convinced of their physical presence in his shadowy bedroom. He thinks of his dreams as real-life experiences, filled with real creatures and people whom he can see, touch, hear, and smell. He supposes also that objects in the outside world — a tree, the moon, an x-ray machine — can have thoughts, feelings, and intentions just as he does (and how menacing an angry x-ray machine could seem to him). In such a fashion, the young child of civilization shares with the primitive a tendency toward animism.

The young child observes that certain actions or events are followed by certain results. He thus begins to grasp the idea of a connection between cause and effect. But he cannot yet understand the process of transformation. That is, he has no way to grasp the idea of a series of changes connecting cause to effect (he sees that a lump of ice melts in the sun, but cannot understand how the heat of the sun transforms ice into water). In his quest for understanding, the three-year-old or four-year-old incessantly asks, "Why?" Even as he asks, however, he constructs his own personal and imaginative theories, and is untroubled if they are unrealistic, illogical, or contradictory.

The young child is learning that people and objects have properties such as color, shape, or size that make them similar to or different from each other. He is learning that objects, sensations, and events can be grouped into categories and classified. However, his understanding of categories is incomplete. He at first concludes that objects belong in the same category if they have one or two similar properties (he observes that a four-legged, furry animal is called a "doggie," and supposes that *all* four-legged furry creatures are dogs even those that meow or moo).

Each such thought characteristic shapes the way a young child is able and likely to think about his body, about his illness, and about the crucial experiences of birth, reproduction, and death.

Body Image

Development of a basic awareness of himself as a distinct and separate physical being is a major developmental accomplishment of the toddler. Early childhood is a period of intense interest in bodily characteristics and concern about physical powers and limitations. It is a time of growing awareness of male or female identity. The totality of the child's ideas, both realistic and imaginary, and his attitudes and emotions about his physical self comprise his body image.

The young child's knowledge of what his body includes is limited to what he has seen, felt, and used — bodily parts, such as eyes, ears, nose, mouth, hair, arms, legs, penis; bodily structures, such as skin and bones; bodily products, such as saliva, blood, urine, stool. He has no way of knowing about most internal structures or organs since he can neither observe them nor feel them in action. For example, young children know from observation that a boy has a penis and testes, but they do not see that a girl has a vagina, uterus, and ovaries. They readily conclude that she is missing an important part, and construct scary theories to account for its lack . . . perhaps it came off or was removed.

The child's knowledge of how his body works is similarly egocentric. For example, since he has no realistic understanding of the female reproductive system, he explains processes such as pregnancy and birth in terms of functions and organs he does know about. Since most things go into the body through the mouth, he theorizes, the pregnant woman must have swallowed a seed. The baby must grow in the "tummy" (with cereal dropping on its head every morning, as one child declared). It must come out through the rear end like a bowel movement, or perhaps through the belly button.

Some young children think of the skin as a body wrapping, like brown paper around a parcel. They imagine that if the skin is punctured or cut the insides might spill out. And so if a knee is scraped or an injection is given, the young child may react in a way that seems excessively fearful to the adult, who sees only a drop or two of blood. The child reacts not to what is really happening but to what he imagines may happen.

The child's ideas about the importance of various bodily parts is also based on personal experience. Many children conclude that the most important parts of their bodies are the ones that have received the most attention. Others believe that all parts are needed to stay alive, and they worry about any interference with the body, perhaps even a haircut.

Body Image and Illness

Health problems affect the child's developing body image in several ways. They may contribute to unrealistic ideas about the body. For example, children who suffered from severe eczema in infancy and whose arms were tied to prevent scratching have been found to portray themselves in drawings as people without arms. Since these children were deprived of continuous experience of their arms as effective, functioning body parts, there had been interference with their developing mental image of the arms. Other children (boys as well as girls) whose abdomens protrude because of enlargement of the liver or spleen, for example, have been observed to imagine themselves pregnant.

Illness may arouse negative feelings about the body. In some conditions, such body products as thick mucus and foul stools may distress and disgust family members (who, after all, have been taught in their own childhood that bad odors are disgusting). Some disorders cause changes in appearance — marked swelling from fluid retention, for example — which may seem grotesque to those who observe the child. The child, sensing these responses, may conclude that his body is disagreeable.

The ill body is at times a source of discomfort rather than of pleasure and accomplishment. It is natural that the child should feel some impatience and anger at his bodily discomfort, and perhaps some sadness.

The young child may lose control over certain bodily functions because of illness. Proud of his recent accomplishment of bowel control, for example, he may unwillingly and helplessly find himself soiling his pants again because of a watery diarrhea. Feeling manly because he can urinate standing up like his father, he may now be required to deposit his urine in a specimen bottle or, worse humiliation, have it taken from him by catheterization. In such ways, his illness deprives him of feelings of mastery.

Theories of Illness

Children strive as actively as adults to grasp the meaning of illness by explaining its cause. In the absence of realistic knowledge about bodily processes, young children construct personal theories of causality.

Having been guided in their behavior by parental approval and disapproval, praise, and punishment, young children commonly develop the belief that badness of thought, word, or action will be followed by a bad experience, namely, a punishment. Therefore, they also reason, if a bad experience (such as illness) occurs, it is probably punishment for wrongdoing.

Because of this sequence of reasoning, most, perhaps all, young children believe that they are to blame for their illness. The child's particular theory will combine what he has heard adults — especially family and doctors — say about him, what he imagines they mean, how he observes they feel about him, and what he has done or thought or wished that he believes to be wrong. A child with diabetes may imagine that he has caused his illness by sneaking too much candy. A child with kidney disease may believe that his illness, especially if there is blood in the urine, was caused by handling his penis.

Most young children also blame outside agents, such as bad

weather, animals, poison, family members. For example, a little girl with heart disease imagined that her brother had caused her illness because, in a tussle, he had hit her on the chest. Not yet capable of logical thought, the young child may quite freely construct different and contradictory theories to explain the same experience.

Concepts of Death

All young children have some experience of death. They have observed it in nature — in insects, fish, other animals. A family friend, a relative, or an older brother's teacher may die. Death is portrayed in story books and dramatized on television — in cartoons, and Westerns, and news about wars and political assassinations. The child's reactions vary according to the personal meaning of the death for him as well as the responses of family members and playmates. A dead beetle may be examined with unfeeling curiosity. Grandfather's death is a time of sadness. An assassination may arouse excitement, horror, and fear: "I don't ever want to be President. Presidents get shot!"

Although death is likely to be emotionally significant to the young child, his understanding of it is quite limited. Defined in terms of adult realism, death is the inevitable, total, and permanent cessation of biological life. (In the view of many, it is also the process of separation of body and soul and the transition to a condition of spiritual afterlife.) The young child is not yet intellectually capable of fully grasping the realistic biological concept.

In the thoughts of a young child, death is temporary. Having little understanding of time, he cannot grasp the idea of permanence. Weeks after the death of a relative he may ask, "When is Grandpa coming back?"

Death is partial. Unable to grasp its totality, the child imagines that only certain functions cease. For example, he may suppose that although the dead one can no longer move or see, he can probably still think or feel. Stillness — or a lack of movement — is frequently equated with death in the child's thoughts. Therefore, if illness interferes with a child's capacity for movement, thoughts of death may readily be aroused.

Death is like sleep. Sleeping creatures lie still with closed eyes. They wake up again. Death must be like that, the child imagines — an idea that is fostered by parents and by children's stories. Adults view this as a comforting and reassuring way of thinking about death. And so it is. Unfortunately, such an idea can also contribute to the young child's anxiety about going to sleep.

Death is connected with angry feelings. A furious six-year-old girl shouts at her mother, "I hate you, I wish you were dead!" A five-year-old boy shrieks at a playmate who squashed his sandcastle, "I'm going to kill you!" A child knows no angrier thing to say. His declarations may relieve him. They may also, however, frighten him. Although adults know the adage that "sticks and stones may break your bones but words will never harm you," young children are not certain that their angry wishes may not come true. Should a relative or friend actually die, especially one at whom the child had sometimes been angry, the child may need active reassurance that his thoughts were not responsible.

Death is punishment. If the child feels that he has been bad and deserves punishment, there may be fearful moments when he expects the worst. If he wishes others to be dead when he is angry at them, why should they not have the same wishes for him? What if their wishes come true?

Death is bodily injury or pain. A little boy who has skinned his knee painfully may sob, "Oh, I'm going to die, I'm going to die," meaning, "My knee hurts badly and I'm afraid it won't ever stop hurting." For him, dying is hurting badly. For the child who is very ill, a central worry is that the doctors won't stop him from hurting. For this he needs reassurance (as well as effective medication).

Death is departure and separation. The child cannot grasp the idea of not-being — "Where was I before I was born?" young children ask urgently. Death must mean being somewhere else — in the churchyard, in heaven. When a beloved relative or pet dies, it is the departure that is the center of distress — a mixture of sadness and of some reproach: "Why did Grandma go away and leave us?" When a young child thinks of his own death, it is the thought "You won't ever see your mommy and daddy again" that is the core of his worry. Parents of critically ill children often sense this even if it is never put into words. They effectively reassure their child just by being near him, perhaps sitting by his bedside and holding his hand.

How Parents Can Help

One of the most crucial developmental tasks for the young child is to begin developing a realistic acceptance of his physical imperfections along with a sense of himself as a worthwhile human being. Parents can foster this process in several ways.

Learn about His Ideas.   Your child can be educated and reassured about his health problem most effectively if you first try to remain aware of his thoughts, worries, and confusions. His ideas are continually developing and changing in response to his advancing intellectual development, as well as his daily physical, social, and emotional experiences. What he imagined last August may be quite different from what he now believes in November.

Young children rarely express their theories in a well-organized way; their minds seem to dart from topic to topic as a hummingbird flits among the flowers. Furthermore, they usually express their ideas most comfortably when talking about someone other than themselves. Therefore, the parent may learn most about the young child's ideas about himself by observing him in play and listening to his running commentary. As Jason puts his teddy bear to bed and declares that teddy is sick, one can quietly interject a few questions: "What made teddy get sick, Jason?" or, "Where does he hurt?"; "What does the sickness do to his tummy?" Jason's answers may reveal much about his theories of the cause, the process, and the effects of his illness.

Offer Corrective Information.   Since what a young child imagines about his illness may be much more worrying than the reality, corrective information can be relieving and reassuring. If Jason declares that his teddy bear is sick because it was a bad boy, it would be helpful to reassure him that "teddy bears don't get sick because they're bad. Boys and girls don't either. Some children are born with a part of their bodies that doesn't work quite right." Or [if the illness was acquired], "Sometimes one part of the body starts making mistakes in doing its job." "Some children have a heart that works too slowly, and they feel tired and out of breath at times."

It is usually most comfortable for the child to listen first to an explanation about a stuffed animal, a doll, or an imaginary child in a story. It may also be more comfortable for you to talk first about the illness of a toy or of an imaginary child. Gradually, as he is ready, your child will recognize the connection between himself and the child in the story. Gradually, as you are ready, you can help him make the connection: "You were born with a heart that works too slowly, too, Jason."

Information is most useful if it is simple, concrete, and related to the child's personal observations and experience. For example, if your child knows about water pumps or gasoline pumps, it might be explained that the heart is a special kind of pump that sends blood flowing through the body. It is helpful to illustrate the explanation with very simple drawings.*

---

*It is worthwhile to ask your child's doctor for help in locating pamphlets describing the illness in simple, layman's language. You might also consult a professional experienced in communicating with young children for help in expressing the information in terms a young child can grasp. Such professionals might include hospital play therapists,

The information you give will be absorbed slowly over a period of time. At first, the child is likely to understand little more than the way his illness makes him feel. For example, four-year-old Ralph, born with cystic fibrosis, would declare, "Bacon and chocolate don't agree with me. They give me tummy aches and make me have too many B.M.'s." Although Ralph could observe the cause-effect relationships between the foods and his tummy aches, only in years to come would he understand the processes involved in foods not "agreeing with" him. However, even such partial understanding gives the child a way of thinking and talking about himself that is somewhat realistic and helps offset feelings of helplessness. It can also make communication with others more comfortable.

Passing through a hospital playroom, a staff social worker paused near Dana who, when he was five, had become blind from an inoperable brain tumor. Feeling a surge of sadness about this little boy's predicament, wishing to reach out and offer comfort, the social worker nonetheless hesitated awkwardly — what can you say to such a child? How can you talk to him?

Sensing her nearness, Dana turned toward her and held out his hand. "Would you help me go across the room to where the blocks are, please? I can't see, you know. I don't want to bump into something." His quiet explanation about his condition made possible a comfortable and spontaneous conversation. Child and social worker found their way across the room together, talking about the block building that Dana was planning.

Accentuate the Positive. Doctors and nurses, understandably enough, tend to direct attention and interest to those bodily parts and functions that don't work properly. Relatives and friends may center their attention on a child's illness. It is important, therefore, in helping your child develop a realistic mental image of himself and a sense of his worth as a human being, to help him recognize what does work properly. Perhaps he does cough a lot because of his cystic fibrosis; however, he can still run, jump, climb, swing, hop, and skip. Perhaps bacon and chocolate don't agree with him; however, lean beef and angel food cake do. Perhaps he does get short of breath because of his heart condition; however, he can still paint vibrantly colored pictures, make up marvelously imaginative stories, and delight all with his sense of humor.

A similar lesson can be taught using your child's observations of others. Young children are keenly interested in differences and similarities between things and people. There are countless opportunities, therefore, to point out that people have many, many different

---

nursery school educators, social group workers, child psychologists, and child psychiatrists.

kinds of imperfections.* As a start, for example, you and your child might notice how many people need eyeglasses because their eyes don't work properly. There are opportunities, furthermore, to point out that all the imperfect people (and who is perfect?) can be kind and loving and helpful and do their jobs well.

Communication Through Language

"We can't communicate," complain troubled couples as they seek counseling. "We're alienated from each other," lament parents and teenagers who seek some words of understanding to bridge the generation gap. "What shall I say?" ask countless worried readers who beseech a popular columnist for catchwords and timely phrases to use in dealing with a myriad of difficulties. All such persons reveal their lack of skill and confidence in using language to express ideas, attitudes, and emotions, and to solve problems.

Effective communication with words has its roots in late infancy and early childhood. The toddler and young child is not only learning the words and phrases of his native language but, equally important, he is learning whether language is a valued and useful channel for self-expression and communication with others. He is learning whether words can be trusted. Therefore, even while his language skills are still limited, he is forming attitudes about language that may influence him throughout his lifetime.

Skill in verbal self-expression is valuable for any child. It may have particular importance for a child with extended illness or disability, especially if he has a reduced capacity for self-expression through bodily activity. It may have particular value for a child who, because of his illness, finds reality frustrating. Skill with words may enable him to release his feelings effectively; it may also provide him with a channel for wish-fulfillment. With verbal skill, his dreams and longings can become the fabric of creativity. The child might learn to spin marvelous tales — as did Robert Louis Stevenson, some of whose poems portrayed memories of prolonged and bleak confinements due to childhood illness. Although few parents will nurture another Stevenson, many can encourage effective self-expression and communication in their children.

*Studies carried out in Great Britain and the United States have shown that 10-12% of all children have some form of significant physical disorder lasting three months or longer.

Fostering Effective Communication

Listening to the Child. A baby's first words are exciting events in his development, and usually command considerable attention from his parents. In fact, their joyful imitation and repetition of his words encourages baby to use them again. It is less easy for parents to respond continuously to the baby's jargon, that is, the long sentences and paragraphs of his expressive but private nonlanguage, or to the flow of the more comprehensible speech that gradually emerges. The stream of chatter may at times seem incessant; the young child's repeated interruptions may at moments be intrusive and annoying. (A young, unmarried social worker, telling the author about a weekend visit from her preschool nephews, wearily exclaimed, "I had no idea children could be so *constant!*") Therefore, parents are apt to tune out much of the child's eager chatter. Although they remain aware of it — as they might of a radio in the background — they pay it little direct attention.

Although it is doubtful that any parent could listen continuously to a young child's flowing communication, it is important not to tune the child out too frequently. Even if you are able to give your child your completely undivided attention for only a few limited periods during the day, such periods can pay rich dividends for parent and child.

Listening is essential in order to know the child's thoughts. An infant's first words have very personal and private meanings. "Ma-ma" may at first mean to the baby the sensations he feels inside when he is hungry and sees someone coming with his bottle. For the toddler, "mommy" is likely to mean you, a special person who exists for the purpose of looking after him. Only in early childhood does he begin to grasp the social or shared meaning of "mommy" — a special classification of woman who has given birth to a child and has a special role in caring for him.

Listening enables you to understand his private meanings and helps him learn the shared meanings. Gradually, for example, you can help him realize that *doggie* does not mean creatures from teddy bears to elephants, as he may first imagine, but rather a particular kind of four-legged, furry animal that barks and wags its tail.

Your attentive listening lets him know that his communications are valued. It conveys concern for his feelings, respect for his ideas, and interest in his imaginings. It enables you to help him clarify the difference between fantasy and reality. His fantasy can be accepted — "That's wonderful make-believe" or, "Wouldn't it be wonderful if we could do that?" — even as you let him know that you understand it is fantasy and not fact.

Talking to the Child about Himself. Children learn language through imitation. Most parents spontaneously say a great deal to the young child about the world he lives in, his behavior, and their attitudes toward his actions. "You musn't touch the stove, it's hot." "Pick up your socks, there's a good boy." "It's been raining out. The grass is wet. You musn't go out or you'll get your shoes all wet and catch a cold." All such comments enrich the child's capacity to give words to his ideas and his actions. However, far fewer parents talk to young children about their feeling states: "You seem sad, Johnny." "I guess you're feeling angry today." "It makes you happy to do that." "I think you are worried about something." When this is done, it helps the young child recognize and identify his emotional experiences and, gradually, learn to express them in words and thus share them with others. Effectiveness in communicating his feelings is one of the most important personal assets a child can develop.

Offering an Example of Clear Communication. Since children do learn their use of language primarily through imitation, not only their vocabulary but also their style of communication will be greatly influenced by your own. Their own capacity to express their emotions directly in words is increased if they observe you to do so: "I feel happy today, John. It's a marvelous day outside." "I'm crabby this afternoon — I guess it's because I'm tired." "I do feel sad because you're sick, Johnny. Sometimes I feel sad enough to cry." Such remarks inform your child that in your family it is fine to express feelings honestly and directly in words.

Children readily notice not only words, however, but also tone of voice, facial expression, the way you hold your body and move around. If the words you use agree with these other messages — if your body is tense, you frown, your voice is harsh, and your words say, "I'm mad!" — children learn that words are reliable and trustworthy. If your words and your other signals disagree, it is puzzling for the child (which message shall he believe?), and he learns that words cannot be trusted.

Communication with the Ill Child

Parents of the child with impaired health may have special difficulty in fostering effective verbal communication. Those parents who are despondent about the disorder, feeling sad, burdened, and weary, may lack the energy to talk much with the child or to listen to him. If the child's own energy level is low because of his illness, his urge to talk may be reduced. If he tends to spend much time alone because of a need for rest or because he lacks energy for and interest in being with others, there may be limited opportunity for verbal communication. Finally, parents may fail to encourage the child to express himself, especially his feelings, because it is so painful for them to be aware that he is sad, worried, or angry about being sick.

If verbal communication between you and your child is limited for any such reasons, you can still help him greatly by recognizing that such a limitation exists and by trying to find out whether the problem arises from his condition or from your own feelings about him. Once the source of the problem is recognized, the solution may be readily available. Possibly your child could spend some time regularly with a trusted relative, friend, or baby-sitter who enjoys talking with young children. Such a person may (because his emotions are less intensely involved than your own) find it easier to listen with interest and sympathy if your child expresses reactions to his illness. Such a person may help him develop verbal skills by reading stories or poems to him, telling make-believe stories, and encouraging him to do the same.

Play

Before doctors were able to identify the rare defect in her metabolism, Polly had lost much of her sight. Watching her small daughter stumble through a world of blurry shapes and outlines, Polly's mother allowed her judgment to become as clouded as the little girl's vision. In a gesture of despair, she gathered up most of Polly's toys one day and added them to a donation of used clothing destined for flood victims: "What use," she grieved, "are toys to Polly now that she can scarcely see them?" And so Polly was deprived of a major way of overcoming the feelings of helplessness and fear her loss of vision aroused.

Gregory had an excess of copper in his system because of another kind of metabolic disorder. His vision was not affected, but he was worried because he seemed unable to control his body. His hands were shaky, his legs felt weak, he often staggered and lost his balance. He was, furthermore, subjected to many difficult studies and tests in the hospital before the doctors could begin to control his disease. Gregory's mother — no less distressed but somewhat wiser than Polly's — designated a corner of the yard as Gregory's "place." There he dug highways, constructed bridges and tunnels; he made his trucks and cars have dreadful collisions until they became totally wrecked, as wrecked as he felt himself to be.

Then Gregory became the fixer. Working patiently for hours, he repaired the vehicles much as the doctors were striving to repair his body. In his mind, Gregory became one of the healers, the powerful ones, and his sense of confidence in himself grew stronger.

Childhood play is often thought of as a pleasant pastime that keeps children out from underfoot: "Run along and play, honey. Mother's busy." Play is fun, but it is also the work of early childhood, and makes major contributions to development.

Play and Learning

Play contributes to the developing body image. Baby's first playthings are his own body and that of his mother. Touching, patting, twisting, and tugging, he enjoys pleasant sensations and expresses natural curiosity. During his infancy, however, his parents are likely to begin limiting the amount of bodily touching, looking, and examining they permit. Through his play with toys, the young child can continue to explore, express and begin to understand the functions of his body in a more acceptable way. He can fill and empty his playthings as he imagines his body is filled (with food) and emptied (of urine and feces). He can cause objects to open and shut as do his eyes, his mouth, and the rings of muscle that close off the urethral and anal openings. His natural impulse to splash and smear his food and bodily products can be acceptably expressed in water play or with clay and finger paint. Furthermore, through the actions of his body in play, the child becomes aware of and enjoys his developing neuromuscular skills such as balance and coordination.

Play also teaches the child about the world around him. It helps him to develop concepts of shape, size, weight, balance, texture, color, and location in space. It helps him learn to recognize similarities and differences.

Play helps the child understand the roles of people in his family and society. In play he can be an imaginary Mom, Dad, Baby, doctor, Good Humor man. He can work out his ideas of who they are and what they do, as well as his ideas of what he may someday become.

Play and Constructive Self-expression

The strong feelings and impulses of childhood seek an outlet. The child is not yet able to deal with them entirely in his thoughts and in words, and cannot always be permitted to express them in direct action. For example, all young children have angry feelings and aggressive impulses. It would be worrying for the child and disagreeable for those around him if he were allowed to hurt himself or others or to destroy property (see Chapter 3). It is much more constructive to encourage release of anger through kicking, punching, hitting, throwing, or hammering the pounding boards, punching bags, balls, and clay that are intended to withstand the assaults of young children. Your child needs such outlets, just as you do (pages 11-13). Similarly, the feelings of pleasure and excitement that surge up need to find expression through jumping, rocking, swinging, dancing, singing, and other forms of joyous play.

The child's play reveals much of his inner world of thought and feeling. Through play a concerned parent can have access to the child's inner experience. There is no better way to learn about the significant events of your child's day than to sit quietly listening to and observing him while he is at play (appease your sense of industry, if you must, by mending socks or shelling peas).

Play and a Sense of Mastery

All of us relive pleasant experiences and come to terms with troubling ones by reviewing them in our thoughts and talking about them to others. Former surgical patients, for example, are renowned for describing their operations to anyone whose attention can be captured. Each time an experience is relived or retold, more feelings can be dispelled. The teller feels less the victim and more the master of the event.

Young children deal with life in similar fashion. They, however, cannot rely only on mental images and words; they need to reenact their experiences through their play. In this way, they repeat their joys, master their fears, and deal with their sense of being small, vulnerable, and at the mercy of events they cannot control or understand. A four-year-old boy, for example, feeling tiny, weak, and helpless after an encounter with an angry giant (his father) can reassure himself by playing the role of jet pilot. As he swoops around the playroom, screeching and roaring like the thundering machine, his imagination allows him to feel some of the skill and knowledge of the pilot as well as the mighty power of the engines.

Play and Illness

For children who must endure difficult medical experiences play can be a significant way of coming to terms with and mastering events that might otherwise be emotionally overwhelming. Play can help prepare the child for a stressful experience such as hospitalization, as well as for a placid aftermath. In his play, the child is the active doer — he is in charge. Like Gregory, he can identify with the powerful ones in his world of experience, and thus feel stronger himself. In his play, the child can alter events to suit his wishes and needs; he can pretend that an event had a different outcome until he is ready to face the outcome it had in reality. In his play, the child can release his fear and anger about the stress in small doses, rather than having his feelings burst out in an explosion that would alarm him and his family.

Because of his illness, the child may need help and encouragement in developing his capacity for play. He may show less initiative than a healthy child in getting started. He may need a companion to arouse his interest in his playthings. Such a companion can only be effective, however, if he or she genuinely enjoys playing with a child. Some adults, including many devoted parents, are quite bored by it.

In planning play experiences for your child, you may wish to consult a nursery school teacher or play therapist about particularly useful play equipment, or you may wish to examine a catalogue from an outstanding manufacturer, such as Creative Playthings or Child Craft. Well-made and imaginative equipment is expensive. Should your budget be limited, such catalogues are also excellent sources of ideas for items that might be produced in a home workshop.

Parents of ill children are often tempted to be particularly permissive about television, which may occupy the child's attention for many hours every day. Television is in some respects a blessing for the shut-in of any age, since it brings the outer world into the homes of those whose opportunities for outside experiences may be limited. On the other hand, television encourages passivity, and children develop and learn most effectively through active experience.

Furthermore, many programs arouse excitement and aggressive impulses in the viewer. A young child has difficulty in understanding and coping with such responses. (One mother reported in dismay that her young son was having erections of his penis whenever he watched intimate love scenes on TV. She asked advice about how to deal with the erections, and was taken aback when she herself was asked, "Why let him watch those programs?") A child already stressed by a bodily disorder may be overloaded by the excitement aroused, especially if he watches TV for prolonged periods.

Widening Social Horizons

The two-year-old, when among other children, can do little more than coexist. Although he may enjoy their company, although he may be interested in watching and trying to imitate their activities, he still has limited capacity for mutual play. The three-year-old, however, can play meaningfully with other children rather than just among them. Such play exposes him to new and varied experiences, sensations, attitudes, and ideas. The development of socialized behavior may be fostered as the child is encouraged to wait for others, to take turns, to control his impulses, to respond to the needs and wishes of other children. The development of realistic thought is fostered as the child exchanges and compares ideas with others, begins to recognize that there are viewpoints different from his own, and begins to understand the shared meanings of words and concepts.

Most young children do have increasing contact with playmates outside the family, within their neighborhoods, in park playgrounds, during visits planned by their mother, or in nursery school programs. To parents of children with impaired health, such contacts may be a source of intense worry.

Worrying Questions

Is He Safe? Allowing a young child to move outside of the orbit of family protection and control is of some concern for most parents. The parent of an ill child may feel intensely worried that the child will be exposed to harmful physical risk. Might he become overly tired or excited? Might his activity result in a fainting spell, a coughing spell? Might he be seriously bruised or cut? Might he catch a cold that would become dangerous?

Will His Differences Be Spotlighted? A child with extended illness does have special physical characteristics that set him apart from a physically healthy child. He may have less energy and become tired sooner. He may need to stop and rest more often because of shortness of breath, coughing, or wheezing. He may need the bathroom more often. He may be susceptible to more serious results from cuts and bruises. He may look different because of pallor, small size, puffiness, or a large abdomen. He may have conspicuous symptoms, such as a cough, a bad odor from his bowel movements, or gas from the intestines. He may need to leave the play group to take his medicine or do his treatment. At a birthday party, he may not be able to share the chocolate cake.

Since the children he plays among are likely to be at the peak of their interest and concern about their own bodily functions, it is natural that they will notice and be curious about your child's special characteristics. They may even feel uneasy about these characteristics because they feel uneasy about their own bodies. They are likely to make comments, ask questions, and perhaps behave in silly ways. Adults who witness such behavior usually think of it as teasing, and comment, "Young children are so cruel." If your own child is the target, you are likely either to feel furious or to want to cry.

Will He Be Avoided?   Parents worry that their child will be avoided, left behind, or left out. If he can't keep up, can't run as fast, gets out of breath, has to stop and rest, will other children want him around? Perhaps they will avoid him because of his symptoms; perhaps their mothers will have told them, "Stay away from Jonathan, he coughs all the time. He must have something catching." (In public places, such as a supermarket, you also may be subject to curious, even accusing, glances, if your child has a conspicuous symptom. It may seem as though people are thinking, "The poor child's sick. Why does she allow him to come out and infect everyone else?")

Helpful Measures

Realistic Protection.   Most young children need supervision while playing together. Their knowledge of risks and consequences is limited; their judgment is unreliable; they place their wishes before those of others; controls over their impulses are uncertain. Young children need to be contained within a playground, yard, or house that is reasonably free of physical hazards and where they are protected against outside dangers. In these respects, the needs of an ill child are little different from those of a healthy child.

However, your child may also have special vulnerabilities to injury or a special susceptibility to infections. In such cases, you may need to establish clear and firm ground rules: play with others only when supervision by a responsible adult or teenager is available; no play with sharp objects; no hitting or throwing things at each other. You may need to ask friends and neighbors to cooperate by keeping their children separated from yours when they seem to be developing a cold.

Decisions about your child's need for physical protection should be made together by you and his doctor. You need the sense of support that comes from knowing that the decision and the sense of risk is shared. You may also need the doctor's support and authority to offset the self-doubts aroused by curious and anxious neighbors and relatives.

Some such decisions are complex and require thoughtful evaluation. They should perhaps be made in a special conference including you, your spouse, and the doctor, without having your child present.*

---

*Some clinics and doctors' offices provide supervised play facilities that children

For example, should a child with cystic fibrosis attend nursery school? The answer would depend on individual and variable factors, including: the doctor's judgment about your child's medical condition; his and your opinion about the benefits a nursery school experience could offer your child; alternatives available for constructive play experiences with other children; personal needs of other family members (mothers of preschool children sometimes desperately need two or three morning periods a week for themselves or for the tranquil care of a young baby).

Encouraging Self-regulation. It has been found that when young children with health problems such as hemophilia sense that their parents consider activity and aggressive behavior dangerous, the children are likely to become outwardly passive and docile. Inwardly, however, they may be seething with unexpressed emotions. Those afflicted children who are encouraged to be active and outgoing, and to express their anger through words and nondestructive physical activity, have been found to begin regulating their activity quite realistically by four or five years of age. They begin to observe the ground rules established by their parents. Being encouraged to exercise some judgments of their own — always with adult opinions readily available to back them up — contributes to their confidence and contentment.

It will probably increase your child's self-assurance among other children if you suggest simple explanations he can make about his special health needs. The explanations can be as simple as those used by Dan'a, "Will you help me find the blocks? I can't see, you know" or by Ralph, "Chocolate doesn't agree with me. It gives me tummy aches." (page 71.)

Seeking Support for Yourself. Because of their parents' worry, many children with impaired health are set apart from others more than their condition actually requires. For example, in one study of children with rheumatic fever, it was found that two thirds of the parents continued or added activity restrictions after the doctor had removed them. Tragically — because it was medically unnecessary — these children were deprived of experiences that encourage constructive self-expression, contribute to self-confidence, and help develop effective relationships with others.

Parents such as these are apt to be labeled "over-protective" and exhorted to stop such behavior. It is scarcely that simple. A sense of risk and apprehension about one's child is difficult to dispel. The symptoms that may result from his activity, even if medically harmless, can be un-

---

can use while their parents talk about "grown-up questions" with the doctor. If there are no such facilities, it is wise to arrange for a separate appointment with the doctor.

pleasant reminders of the illness. The remarks, questions, or teasing of playmates confront him and you with repeated and disagreeable reminders that your child does have a disorder that you long occasionally to put out of your thoughts.

Since it is natural to wish to shelter your child — and yourself — from such confrontations, you may need considerable support in exposing him — and yourself — to them. Not only is it helpful to share your decisions about how much exposure to encourage, but it is also comforting to share your worry with an understanding friend or relative. Sharing your worry may enable you to endure it.

Hospitalization

A doctor who understood physical disease considerably better than the mental and emotional development of young children frequently expressed perplexity when nurses described the unhappiness of his young patients during the first hours after their admission to the hospital. "But we haven't *done* anything to the child yet," he would remark, revealing that he shared a widespread misconception that it is only the medical procedures that are stressful to young hospitalized children. In actuality, there are several important sources of stress. Understanding these can enable parents as well as the staff help the child cope with them more effectively.

Sources of Stress

The Sense of Misery.   A child needing hospitalization usually feels sick, and his physical misery is a primary source of stress. Unfortunately, the stress may also be intensified by his ideas and feelings about his physical ailments. There is a fragile separation between fact and fancy in the thoughts of the young child. Under the stress of physical misery, this separation may break down. The mind may be swamped by unpleasant fancies. A common fancy is one expressed by Nancy, a three-and-a-half-year-old who listened intently during a clinic visit as her mother and doctor discussed plans for her hospital admission. After her return home from the clinic, Nancy became unusually sweet, affectionate, and ingratiating toward her mother. "Mommy," she declared, "I'm going to be very good, and then I won't have to go to the hospital." Nancy revealed the belief common in early childhood that physical misery and hospitalization are consequences of being bad. Such a belief, accompanied by a sense of badness and of guilt, colors the child's experience with emotional misery.

Separation.   To the infant, when mother is absent it is as though she has ceased to exist. The young child has begun to understand that his mother has an existence apart from his own. He still, however, thinks of her primarily in terms of his own needs and wishes. When he needs her comfort and reassurance, his capacity to wait is limited. Furthermore, he still lacks the realistic sense of time that helps an older child endure separation.

The child constructs theories to account for his mother's absence. Such theories are apt to be unrealistic, especially if the child has not been adequately prepared for the separation. Since he views parents as all-powerful, he readily supposes that they must have *wanted* to leave him, rather than that they *had* to leave him. He readily imagines that they wanted to leave him because he was bad or unlovable.

Separation from mother, therefore, arouses fears of abandonment in the hospitalized child (as it does for different reasons in the infant and toddler*). It may become the most urgent source of anxiety, even in a child who normally copes well with periods of separation. If parental visiting is extremely limited, the child must devote much of his energy to trying to suppress his feelings of having been deserted.

Loss of Control.   His accomplishments in controlling his body and regulating his behavior are a source of pride and confidence to the young child. In the hospital, many of his accomplishments may be ignored. He may find he is treated "like a baby," being washed, fed, dressed, and denied the use of a toilet. He may even suffer the indignity of sleeping in a bed with railings that seems like a crib. He may lose his own controls over bodily functions by vomiting, wetting the bed, having diarrhea. Regulation of his behavior, based on newfound capacities to delay, think about his actions, recall the past, anticipate the future, may break down under stress, and he may indulge himself in bouts of crying, shouting, hitting, or throwing that trouble him as much as those around him.

Fear of Bodily Harm.   Bodily manipulations and the physical procedures involved in medical and nursing care are apt to be more worrying for the young child than for the infant and toddler. In fact, there are several reasons — in addition to the reality of having a sick body — why young children may feel intense anxiety about the well-being of their bodies. First, the child's sense of his physical self, his body image, is newly developed and still quite uncertain. The child does not understand the structures and functions of his body; he does not yet feel confidence in its intactness. Second, he observes that the bodies of some others are different from his, and wonders if such changes could occur to himself as well. (There are few sights more worrying to a four-year-old

*See Chapter 3.

boy than that of an amputee without a prosthesis collecting money for a veterans' organization.) Third, when he has sought comfort or pleasure from his own body — sucking his thumb, caressing his hair, holding his genitals — he may have been admonished, "Don't do that; that's not nice." In fact, some parents are so troubled about witnessing a child handle his genitals that they threaten, "If you do that, it'll fall off!" or, more frightening, "I'll cut it off!"

Fourth, his developing conscience — the sense of goodness and badness, right and wrong — leads him to expect punishment for his bad thoughts or feelings. He readily supposes that such punishment may take the form of bodily hurt. Fifth, he still believes that inanimate objects can have thoughts, feelings, and intentions just as he does. Therefore, the diagnostic apparatus and therapeutic equipment in a hospital can seem very scary indeed. After all, an angry x-ray machine might crush him, might it not?

Restraint of Movement.   Movement is no less important for the child than for the infant (Chapter 3). It offers pleasure, releases tension, communicates need, expresses emotion, promotes learning, enhances a sense of mastery, contributes to the growing sense of individuality and independence, and provides social experience. The hospital environment, medical procedures, or the illness itself may result in restriction of movement. Not only is the child then deprived of a major channel for self-expression, but this restraint may divert his attention from the world around him and focus it exclusively on his body and his inner world of fear and fancy.

Memory of Previous Hospitalizations.   His developing intellectual capacities enable the young child to store memories that can be a source of comfort or of apprehension. If an earlier hospitalization involved painful and frightening experiences, it is likely that the child's fear of a current hospitalization will be intensified by his memories. Unfortunately, the opposite is not necessarily true. Even if an earlier stress was successfully mastered, the child's advancing development may have brought new apprehensions to the fore.

The stresses of hospitalization arise, therefore, only in part from the physical illness and its treatment. They also arise from his ideas and his feelings about the events and sensations that he experiences.

Reactions to Stress

The hospitalized child may respond to these stresses with a variety of changes in his personality, his behavior, and his relations to others. Many such changes are temporary and serve a useful purpose in helping the child cope with the experience.

Regression. The child may backslide in his development. Recent accomplishments in behavior and self-regulation may be lost, and he may appear more babyish than usual. He may show increased whining, clinging, crying, thumbsucking, and baby talk. He may indulge in snatching, hitting, throwing, kicking. He may wet the bed and soil himself. As the understanding young mother of a three-year-old observed, "It's Lisa's way of telling us that she's still a baby, and she doesn't feel grown up enough to be in the hospital." Unfortunately, such backsliding can be alarming to parents who fail to understand its meaning.

Withdrawal. The child may become absorbed in himself and his body. He may seem indifferent and unresponsive to those around him. Such withdrawal, often seen in acute illness, may be helpful in allowing the child to conserve energy for recovery. It may also, of course, be a response to medication he has been given. His apathy and unresponsiveness are, however, saddening and worrying for his parents.

Compliance. The child may become strikingly docile and compliant — too good. Such children may win the approval of hospital staff because they are easy and pleasant to care for, but, unfortunately, children who behave thus may be feeling overwhelmed. Furthermore, tremendous energy must be used by the child to keep his emotions and behavior under restraint. The suppressed feelings will insistently seek an outlet.

Philip, age three-and-a-half, experienced a two-week hospitalization in which it was necessary to draw blood samples from his veins, including the jugular vein in his neck, several times each day. The first time this was done, Philip, as one would expect, cried and struggled. To insure his physical safety, he was surrounded by staff who held him motionless. Thereafter, Philip struggled less and less each time. He became passive and yielding, and even gave up the protest of tears. In between procedures, he seemed quiet and content.

After his return home, however, his mother became alarmed. His house was located quite near a state highway frequently traveled by large trucks. Each time he heard a truck, Philip would momentarily stiffen, and then begin to scream in panic. He trembled for 10–15 minutes after the truck had passed.

Philip's mother sought the advice of a social worker who had been concerned about Philip's adjustment in the hospital. While discussing the problem, the mother, who had spent most of each day in the hospital with him, remembered that to divert the boy during her visits she had often walked with him to a hospital window through which they could watch and hear trucks at work on a construction project. Clearly, the sound of trucks at home was the cue that was flooding Philip's mind with fearful memories and suppressed feelings connected with hospitalization.

Recognizing the link, his mother encouraged the child actively to discharge his pent-up feelings in words and in play. During the next several weeks, Philip's stuffed animals, his parents, and their visitors were subjected to hundreds of injections with Philip's toy syringe. Gradually his anxiety seemed to be dispelled.

Protest.   In contrast to Philip, another young child may react with aggressive and protesting behavior. He may oppose every procedure with physical struggles, have outbursts of temper, and heap angry verbal abuse on his caretakers. Understandable as such outbursts are, unrestrained aggressive behavior may actually work against the child's best interests. First, such behavior usually arouses resentment, anger, and dislike within the staff, which the child will sense and which will interfere with effective care. Second, unrestrained aggression will probably arouse guilt and anxiety within the child himself. Third, his anger and abuse will be extremely distressing to his parents — already feeling regretful and perhaps guilty about the hospitalization — and may lead them to reduce their visiting.

Other Responses.   Regression, withdrawal, compliance, and protest are observed among infants as well as among young children. In early childhood, new ways of dealing with stress are observed also. For example, unendurable thoughts and feelings may be completely eliminated from the child's awareness. There will be denial on the child's part that he is sick at all, that he needs to be hospitalized, or that he even cares. Alternately, he may seem to accept his situation, but talk about it in a way that is curiously devoid of emotion. The ideas, in such instances, have been isolated from the feelings surrounding them. Or, if the emotions are too intense to endure, the child may project them on others. For example, if his own anger is too scary, he may imagine that he is not angry at all but that others have very hostile feelings toward him. This is scary also but more acceptable to him. The child may deal with his feelings of helplessness and vulnerability by imagining himself to be one of the strong and powerful adults around him — perhaps a doctor or nurse. He may try to help them do their work, imitate them in his play, wear a nurse's cap or a stethoscope as a symbol of the strength he seeks.

Many of the child's own responses and behavioral strategies help him to endure hospitalization. However, parents and staff, working in collaboration, can find many additional ways to help him. When a child is able to master such a difficult experience, considerable mental and emotional growth often result.

Helpful Measures

Preparation.   A young child can be helped to begin coping with a difficult experience even before it occurs through the process of preparation. Preparation starts with imparting simple, concrete information about what the child is going to feel and observe and about why the experience will take place. The information is most wisely given in small doses, dealing first with the questions which are most urgent for the child. For example, before hospitalization the most important information may concern the fact that he will stay in the hospital overnight, that mother will (or won't) stay with him, that he will be in his own room (or with other children), that he will sleep in a special, high bed, that nurses will help him with his clothes, meals, washing, and going to the bathroom, and that the doctor (or doctors) will examine him and decide what special care he needs. He will need reassurance that he isn't going to the hospital because he's done something wrong, but because his doctor believes it is needed to help him feel better.

It will be difficult for you to prepare your child constructively if you are, yourself, intensely fearful about the hospitalization. (Fear is communicated not only in words, but also in your facial expression, your tone of voice, your way of moving and of holding your child.) Furthermore, you can explain to your child only what you understand. Therefore, the first step is to prepare yourself. It is helpful to talk over your fears and questions with the doctor. It is helpful to find out (from him or from the hospital admitting office) about hospital policies that will influence your child's comfort: for example, visiting hours, living-in facilities for parents, and such details as whether your child can bring his own nightclothes and a special comforter — perhaps a security blanket or a stuffed animal.

It may be most comfortable and effective for you to introduce the idea of hospitalization to your child indirectly. You might read him a story about going to the hospital, or tell him your own story, using simple drawings as illustrations. You might carry out some playacting with a doll, puppet, or stuffed animal: "Teddy's cough has been bothering him a lot. The doctor thinks he should go to the hospital so that they can try some special medicines to help him feel better." After explaining about the teddy bear, it may be easier to say, "Dr. Jones thinks that would be a good idea for you, too, Jimmy."

Such information will need to be repeated several times since the young child can only absorb it slowly.

Joanne, a bright four-year-old, was taken on a preparatory visit through the children's division where she was to be hospitalized. She was accompanied by her mother and the social worker, who also introduced her to the friendly head nurse. Joanne was shown the room she would stay in, allowed to crank the bed she would sleep in, investigate the closet and dresser, explore the playroom, examine some toys and use the bathroom. Back in the social worker's office, the mother asked Joanne what she had thought of it all. "It's nice," said Joanne politely, "but when *I* come to the hospital, where will *I* stay — over in Dr. Brown's place [office]?" Clearly, the task of preparation had scarcely begun.

Preparation should include opportunity for the child to reveal what he has or has not understood. Joanne did not connect with herself what she had observed; Nancy (page 82) imagined that she could avoid hospitalization if she was very good.

Preparation should include opportunities for the child to release feelings about the approaching experience. In fact, he may not be able to absorb much information until his feelings have been released; apprehension blocks understanding among children as well as among adults. This release of feeling may afford the child one of the greatest emotional benefits of preparation. His excitement, fear, anger, and sadness about hospitalization can gradually be discharged in small amounts that the child can tolerate, rather than be suppressed or come out in huge and frightening outbursts. Unfortunately, the child's release of feeling can be extremely uncomfortable for parents; it is very painful indeed to hear your child reproach you angrily or cry fearfully when you already feel worried, sad, and regretful about hospitalization. It is sufficiently uncomfortable so that many parents try to avoid preparation altogether: "It's better not to tell him, he would just get upset." Understandable as this position is, it is usually not helpful to the child. It is far more constructive to recognize that you will need support from family, friends, or professional persons in enduring your child's distress, and to seek such support in advance. It is also constructive to encourage your child to work out his feelings through active play rather than through upsetting encounters with you (although some encounters are inevitable).

Preparation should include reassurance that the child will be helped to cope with the experience. He needs to know that his parents will be with him at certain times. He needs to know that his mother or his doctor or nurse will try to find out and explain to him each day what is going to happen. He needs help in knowing how he can take an active part in his own care. A child with cystic fibrosis, being prepared to sleep in a mist tent, expressed intense fear that he would be unable to get out and that his mother wouldn't hear him if he called. His mother and the inhalation therapist wisely showed him how he could crawl under the tent, and then allowed him to practice doing this many times before he was expected to settle down for the night.

Ideally, perhaps, preparation should be started only a few days before the hospital admission. Unfortunately, the timing may not be optional. If the child is acutely ill, admission may be urgent and sudden. Or a child may learn of a planned hospitalization quite far in advance. Conversation about it may be overheard in the doctor's office or at home, or the child may become aware from a parent's tense and worried manner that something is in the air. Should the child thus learn or sense that an unknown but scary event is planned, his mind may become swamped by frightening fantasies unless the reality is brought into the open.

Preparation should continue, step by step, through the entire hospitalization and until the child has returned home. Many parents need information and guidance from professional persons in beginning the preparation process with their child. Ask the child's doctor or the hospital admissions office whether there is a special nurse, social worker, or play therapist on the staff who can guide and work with you in preparing your child effectively. Pamphlets containing helpful information are available in many larger medical centers.

Welcome as the discharge from the hospital usually is, preparation is also needed for the return home. The child may need help in understanding that he will not necessarily be restored to complete health and that special treatments and medicines may need to continue. Parents need to develop confidence that they have the knowledge and the skill to meet his special needs; they need opportunities to seek instruction and guidance from appropriate members of the hospital staff. Furthermore, they need to prepare themselves for the fact that the child is likely to show some alterations in his behavior for several weeks or even months. When he is later faced with a new experience — starting kindergarten for example — the prospect of another separation from his parents may reawaken anxieties connected with hospitalization, and the intensity of his reactions may puzzle his parents unless they are able to understand the connection.

Visiting. Most young children, in the usual course of daily life, deal successfully with separations from their parents. The hospitalized child, however, is likely to feel an increased need for their presence because of the stresses he is experiencing. His parents may feel as emotionally torn about visiting as the parents of the infant and toddler (Chapter 3). Although they may wholeheartedly wish to be with their child to comfort and reassure him, they may also find his physical and emotional misery unbearable; they may find the hospital environment strange and frightening; they may feel concerned about the needs of other family members at home.

For these reasons, some parents feel unable to spend the entire day with their child or to stay overnight, even if hospital regulations permit. However, children benefit greatly even from visiting that is limited, especially if visits are planned with them and are predictable. Since the child's sense of time is quite uncertain, it is helpful if plans are clear and specific: when John wakes up after the operation, Mommy (Daddy) will be there; Mommy (Daddy) will be there to help him get ready for the night; Mommy (Daddy) will come at lunchtime. If you are unable to make specific plans for your return before you leave him, it is helpful to explain that you will telephone his nurse and ask her to tell him when you are coming back.

It is supportive if at least one parent can visit every day. The child can be helped to endure the intervals between visits by other links with home — a favorite stuffed animal or security blanket, a photograph of the family pet, a drawing sent by brother or sister, even a phone conversation with you if regulations permit. Although such reminders may bring sadness, the flow of tears that may follow can be healing.

Promoting Trust in the Staff. The child is likely to tolerate separation more successfully if he has confidence in the hospital staff. You can scarcely enhance his feeling of trust unless you have confidence in the staff yourself. Apprehensive parents are likely to feel critical and to find fault with staff members; parents (especially mothers) feeling guilty and helpless about the illness are prone to feel that the nurses are usurping their role with the child.

Thoughtful discussion of such feelings, perhaps with a nonmedical professional person, such as the hospital social worker or chaplain, often helps one to understand and dispel them. It may also help if you seek ways of collaborating actively with the staff in caring for your child. For example, if you share your concerns with them, you may begin to sense their own interest and concern for your child and for you. If you share your observations of your child's personality and behavior at home, they may share their observations of his responses in the hospital. Together, you and they can plan ways in which you can participate in his care, perhaps helping him bathe and dress, sharing meals, taking him for a walk, reading a story. Together you and they can plan visiting times and prepare him for the sadness of your departure and the joy of your return.

Most hospital personnel have chosen their professions out of a personal need and desire to help and to heal. Staff members are likely to find the care of your child more deeply satisfying, and to carry it out more effectively, if they sense that they really matter to him and that you value their help.

Permitting Release of Feeling. It is natural for a child to feel frightened, angry, and sad about being in the hospital. The child may need encouragement to express such feelings, in words and in tears, to a trusted person, his parent, a kind nurse, a friendly doctor. If possible, this should occur in private, so that the child's outburst of misery does not distress the other patients and their parents.

Although the child needs opportunity to express anger, he also needs reassurance that aggressive attacks that might hurt others or destroy property will not be allowed. As has been mentioned, should a child's expressions of rage be uncontrolled, it is almost certain both that he will become anxious and guilty and that he will provoke the staff's dislike.

Encouraging Play. It is helpful if emotional release can be experienced through active play also. Many hospitals have playrooms and play programs supervised by nursery school teachers, play therapists, special nurses, or social group workers. In such play, children can increase their sense of mastery by enacting the roles of doctor, nurse, or parent — and imagining themselves as being one of the powerful ones for a short while. They can derive encouragement from seeing other children who are coping successfully with illness (although they do need reassurance that the ailments of the others will not befall them also). Feelings of aloneness may be replaced by a sense of kinship — "we're all in the same boat together." The play program will be fun and offer pleasant experiences to offset others that are disagreeable. The program helps to organize the hours in each endless day, and prevents the child from withdrawing totally into his inner world of fear and fancy.

Encouraging Self-care. Although the hospitalized child needs to know that others will give him the care he requires, he may feel less anxious if the many things he can still do for himself are pointed out. For example, if allowed, he might wash his own face, help collect his own urine specimen, hold a towel for the nurse, crank his own bed, change his clothes. If his condition permits, he might have meals at a table in the playroom rather than in bed, and might cut up his own potatoes. He might feel more his own man in blue jeans and a baseball shirt than in pajamas. If parents and staff can agree that self-mastery is a valuable goal for the ill child, they show remarkable ingenuity in helping the child move toward that goal.

5

Coping with Impaired Health in Mid-childhood

Being Different

"But Mom, *nobody* wears rubbers like that to school any more! Do you want the kids to think I'm *queer*?" Such pleas symbolize one of the most important characteristics of mid-childhood: the mounting need to be the same as "the kids" and to be accepted by them.

Peer Groups — How and Why

After he reaches school age, an increasing proportion of a child's experience usually takes place outside his home. He comes into association with other youngsters in school, in the neighborhood, in activities such as Scouts and team sports. These youngsters tend to form themselves into groups that share enough common characteristics to be thought of as peer groups. Such associations influence and contribute to a child's development in important ways.

As the child strives to gain increasing independence from his parents, he strongly needs a sense of belonging. A feeling of kinship with his peers gives the child some emotional support, although girls and boys may seek it in somewhat different ways.

The group associations of girls may be quite variable in nature. Girls are often expected, even encouraged, to maintain a closer attachment to their mothers than boys are usually permitted, and so girls may have a somewhat less urgent need for group or "gang" membership. They may associate in smaller groups, perhaps intimate twosomes or threesomes. They may mingle at the fringes of the male group, either as interested onlookers or hoping to be accepted as members.

For boys, however, the gang is an extremely important proving ground. The support of "the guys" helps a boy quell his occasional wishes for dependency on and closeness to his mother; it helps him deny any envy of girls (who are allowed to be openly dependent). The gang joins him in derogating girls and calling them "sissies." In fact, group support and recognition of his masculine independence may be crucially important for the boy with a health problem, since his illness may necessitate a more passive and dependent relationship with his mother than he can comfortably accept.

In addition to fostering independence from their parents, kinship with their peers helps youngsters develop a more secure sense of their identities as boy-becoming-man and girl-becoming-woman. Their natural interest in the structures, functions, and sensations of their male or female bodies can be shared with peers. Youngsters can derive reassurance from realizing that the others also have a natural tendency to reduce tension by seeking comfort from their bodies — stroking their hair, nibbling their fingers, handling their genitals. Within the peer group, appropriate interest in sexuality is shared: this is the age of secrets, dirty words, sexual jokes and gestures, often repeated with glee whether or not they are understood.

Affectionate relationships are established. The earlier, intensely tender and loving attachment to the parents (Chapter 4) has been largely renounced and forgotten. However, these feelings seek new objects. In the peer group, the child can make a gradual transition from attachment to the parents, moving through the way station of affectionate bonds with others like himself (usually youngsters of the same sex) toward the ultimate interest in members of the opposite sex and in choosing a mate.

Because his peers are crucially important to the child, their opinions can have a major influence on his self-esteem. At home, in a normally devoted family, he has been loved and valued as a family member just because he exists. Among his peers (and the adults associated with them, such as teachers, coaches, or Scout leaders), the child is valued for what he achieves. At home, he was judged and treated as an individual with particular significance to his family. Among his peers, the child is judged as a member of a group, in relation to collective standards of behavior, such as being loyal, not "snitching," taking a dare. He may take a certain position as leader or follower, and be expected to carry out certain responsibilities. In the long run, the judgments and opinions of his peers may help the child develop a more realistic conception of himself than he would develop within his family alone.

Because he is striving to gain independence from his family, the child may cling desperately to group norms of conduct, achievement, and appearance. His compliance may be indiscriminate — to prove his courage, he may accept a dare to shoplift or cheat on a test as readily as a challenge to skate on thawing ice.* He may become the clown and subject himself to ridicule rather than risk being ignored.

In time, most children do develop compassion, feelings of empathy for others, and tolerance for individuality (a child with a disability may

---

*And he may also be deeply relieved if he is discovered by his parents, and they make it very clear that such actions are unacceptable within their family value system.

come to be protected, and perhaps given a special position as group mascot). However, the need for conformity is, for a while, intense, probably reaching a peak between 10 and 12 years of age, in fifth and sixth grades. During this period, group expectations and judgments can be harsh. All children, healthy as well as ill, experience moments of anguish when they feel they deviate or fail to measure up.

Their distress may be intensified because the approach of adolescence is typically heralded by increasing feelings of inner uncertainty: "Who am I?" "Who do I like?" "Who do I want as my friend?" "Who wants me as his friend?" This is a time when the composition of peer groups may undergo rapid, bewildering shifts. Children who are devoted friends one week become mortal enemies the next. Devoted parents of all children, healthy or ill, are witness to their children's emotional pain in this turbulent period, and suffer with them.

Difference Is a Reality

"You know, Mom, I'm not normal," declared a 10-year-old boy with mild asthma, when "shooting baskets" had triggered a coughing spell. His simple statement, which caused his mother a momentary feeling of shock and sadness, reflected that he had a more realistic view of himself than she had achieved.

A child with a health problem *is* different. His appearance may be changed either by the disorder itself or by the medical treatment he receives. The differences are observed by his peers; they are interpreted or misinterpreted and commented on according to their attitudes and level of understanding. He may be unusually short ("shrimp," "runt"). He may look puffy because his tissues hold excess fluid ("fatty"). An enlarged organ may cause the abdomen to protrude ("Patty's going to have a baby"). He may be pale, have bluish lips, scanty hair, or some deformities of joints or limbs.

Even if his appearance is normal, the child's physical functions may be obviously different. He may tire quickly, become short of breath, have fainting or shaky spells, spasms of coughing. He may become nauseated, or need to urinate or defecate frequently. His bowel movements may have an unusually foul odor, or he may have excess gas from the intestines. He may easily develop swellings or severe bruises after a bump.

Your child's disorder may necessitate a special diet that makes him feel conspicuous in the school lunchroom or at group gatherings or parties. He may have to interrupt his activities to take pills at regular times, to have an injection, or to carry out a special procedure of physiotherapy or inhalation therapy. His medicine may even alter his mood or make him feel drowsy.

Your child's disorder may cause prolonged or recurrent discomfort or pain that may drain away his energy, make him irritable or sad and, naturally, influence the way he behaves.

All such differences will, inevitably, be noticed by his peers. In their own struggle for conformity and acceptance, differences may make them uneasy, embarrassed, and apparently unsympathetic. In their own efforts to subdue and react against their earlier impulses to mess, soil, or smear, they may show an exaggerated disgust at "gross" manifestations of illness, such as mucus or flatulence. Furthermore, their attitudes toward your child will be influenced by their own families and ethnic background. Lamentably, in some ethnic groups there is still considerable aversion — fear and hostility — to illness or bodily distortion, which is viewed as a sign of evil in the afflicted person.

Concealment versus Disclosure

A child with a physical disorder worries about how his peers will react to the fact that he is different. Basically he fears rejection, although his fear may be expressed in a variety of ways.* He may imagine that the kids will think he's "weird," a "Martian," a "freak." He fears that they will tease him, pick on him, talk about him. Boys approaching puberty (10- and 11-year-olds) may have heightened concern about their manliness. "The kids will think you're a weakling." "In track, you've got to stop and cough. You can't take it." "You wouldn't be worthy of your friends. You couldn't belong to a strong gang because you couldn't hold your own in a fight." Such fears are common among children with many different health impairments.

Although afflicted children wish that their disorders could remain hidden to avoid possible rejection by their peers, this wish may be paralleled by an intense longing to share the "secret," to confide in a trusted friend. A nine-year-old-boy explained that after he told a friend, "I felt good inside. I was always trying to keep it in, and then all of a sudden it just busted out." An 11-year-old-boy thought that one would *want* to tell a special friend "because he doesn't, you know, want to keep it in all his life."

The experience of confiding in a trusted friend, and then realizing

*Examples are drawn from an unpublished study of school-age boys carried out in the Yale Cystic Fibrosis Program. This study was initiated by Bruce Axelrod, M.D., a "resident" in pediatrics. The study was designed and carried out by Dr. Axelrod and the author. Dr. Axelrod is currently acting assistant professor of pediatrics and psychiatry, University of Washington School of Medicine.

that he is still accepted and valued in spite of his disorder, is deeply meaningful and reassuring for a child. But telling the secret is also a testing out of his acceptability. The child senses that he is putting himself on the line, and so it is an exposure he thinks about with considerable apprehension.

Helpful Measures

Revealing the Disorder. Parents sometimes try to protect their children from hurt by encouraging them to try to hide their symptoms or their medicine: "Don't let the kids in school see you taking your pills." Unfortunately, such concealment rarely works, and it encourages the child to believe that his disorder is a shameful secret.

On the other hand, it is not helpful if your child blurts out information in a way that makes his peers feel intensely uncomfortable. For example, a 10-year-old boy would repeatedly show his pills to his schoolmates and volunteer, "I got to take these to stay alive." "No kidding, Ralph?" other youngsters would say, in shocked disbelief. "That's right," Ralph would declare. "If I don't take them I'm going to die." Ralph's rather aggressive revelations (which were not quite accurate anyway) forced information on his peers that aroused great anxiety, and although it gained him momentary attention, the other youngsters tended to avoid him when possible.

It may be helpful for you and your child to think up and even rehearse a few simple explanations about his disorder which he might offer his peers. For example, an 11-year-old girl with an intestinal disorder told her friends, "I have a problem with my bowels, and if I don't take special pills I get bad cramps." It is helpful to point out to your child that although some youngsters will accept the disclosure in a matter-of-fact way, others may react with embarrassment or even disgust. If your child can tolerate this, perhaps even adding to his explanation a comment like, "Gross, isn't it?", his peers are likely to become accepting and sympathetic.

If other youngsters avoid or tease a child, it is natural for his parents to sympathize with him, to feel angry, and to blame the other youngsters. It is more helpful to your child, however, to point out that physical differences do tend to make kids his age feel uneasy, but that this feeling usually lasts only a short while. If your child can put up with it for a while (with your sympathetic support), the gang will usually begin to rally around.* One lad described such an experience in relation

---

*If your child is subjected to prolonged teasing or ridicule, or is constantly avoided by others, something is probably awry in the way he presents himself to them. Try to make

to the problem of keeping up with others on his bike: "I was pretty slow and my bike was old. They were going uphill and I couldn't keep up with them. I told them, 'I have a problem with my lungs, and it makes me tired, you know. I just can't keep up with you, so you'll have to take a slower pace,' and, you know, I felt good inside because they did slow down."

Although some exposure of the child's special physical condition is inevitable, it is tactful to avoid unnecessary exposure. For example, parents whose child sleeps in a mist tent may choose to put the tent away during the daytime so their child does not continually have to deal with his playmates' questions and reactions. However, if a friend is expected to "sleep over," the parent would need to help the child rehearse some simple explanations about the tent.

Offering Activity Guidelines. The school-age child may find it more difficult than the preschooler to maintain a level of activity that keeps him physically comfortable since the esteem of his peers is so important to him. A boy has a special need to prove himself on the testing ground of physical skills, and is concerned about being considered worthy of his group. It is important, therefore, to offer guidelines that are as clear as possible, and to encourage him to draw on outside authority when he must limit his activity. He is less likely to feel that he is showing he "can't take it" if he can say, "It's a rule that I'm supposed to stop and rest five minutes when I start to wheeze." And since it is harder to say, "My mother told me" than to refer to the guidance of his doctor, it helps him if you ask the doctor to discuss activity guidelines directly with your child as well as with you.

Coping with Difference at School. In mid-childhood, classmates are one of the most significant peer groups. Helping the child deal successfully with his disorder in school requires the active cooperation of parent, principal, teachers (including physical education teachers) and school nurse. Many parents attempt to conceal their child's condition from the school staff, fearing that knowledge of it might somehow arouse negative, pitying, preferential, or discriminatory attitudes and treatment of the child.

In reality, the opposite is normally the case. The school staff will, without accurate information, be forced to make their own interpretations of what they observe. These interpretations, perhaps based on what is imagined or rumored about the child's disorder, may be incorrect and lead to unrealistic expectations. For example, teachers sometimes

---

your own observations about what is going wrong. Then it may be valuable to seek professional guidance to help your child establish satisfying relationships.

mistakenly suppose that children with certain chronic illnesses are likely to be intellectually dull. Therefore, they may expect an inappropriately low level of performance from the child.

If the child should manifest a learning problem, it may mistakenly be attributed to his disorder. Other — remedial — conditions that are actually causing the difficulty may be overlooked. For example, one little girl had persistent difficulty with copying tasks requiring coordination between what her eyes perceived and what movements her hand then made. For two years, she experienced failure and discouragement because her teachers concluded that this must be an untreatable manifestation of her physical disorder. Only when it was determined that she had a mild "visuomotor handicap," unrelated to her blood disease, was she given the special remedial help that enabled her to gain a sense of accomplishment.

Children with chronic illness are sometimes smaller than average. Because of this, teachers (and others) may tend to perceive them as being younger than their actual age, and respond accordingly.

It is in your child's best interests to inform the school about his health impairment and whether it is expected to have any influence on his learning capacities. This is most effectively done in a personal conference. Since records are not always kept or reexamined as carefully as you might wish, it is important to review your child's status every year with his current teachers. If your child's disorder is a rare one, it would be helpful to offer the staff a pamphlet which describes the condition accurately and clearly. (Voluntary health agencies distribute such pamphlets.)

Having established channels of communication about your child, you will then be able to work cooperatively to meet his needs in school and reduce his sense of being different. For example, although pleasant in one sense to be "teacher's pet," it burdens a child with the resentment of his classmates. If the teacher's expectations are realistic, he or she may feel less need to favor or pamper your child. Teachers could foster understanding and acceptance of your child's needs by including some discussion of significant medical problems in the health or science curriculum. You and the teachers may be able to anticipate some of your child's necessary absences from school, and plan for special home assignments or tutorial help so that your child won't be conspicuously out of step with the academic pace of his classroom. (In many communities, a prolonged absence is required before the pupil is eligible for homebound teaching. Short, frequent absences are usually not provided for.)

You and the staff could plan together to meet the child's special physical needs. If he is short winded or lacking stamina, and the distances between classrooms are great or involve stair climbing, his schedule might be adjusted to allow for this. If he has frequent need for the bathroom, it might be arranged with his teacher for him to leave the classroom unobtrusively. If his stools have a particularly foul odor, he might be permitted to use the bathroom near the nurse's office. (She can cope with the odor afterward — either with a spray or by burning a wooden match — far more readily than he can cope with his classmates' expressions of disgust.) Arrangements might be made for unobtrusive but supervised taking of medication (a particularly sensitive problem nowadays, since drug abuse has led to stringent restrictions about pill taking in many school districts). His physical education program might be modified to encourage appropriate activity while avoiding stresses beyond his physical capacities. If he is conspicuously underweight or underdeveloped, nonessential bodily exposure in the shower room might be avoided.

Identifying with Others.   The school-age child strives to develop a sense of kinship with others like himself. A child with a physical disorder may profit from being helped to recognize other children in his school and community with physical disabilities, who must deal with many problems similar to those he faces.

When the child is able to cope with overnight separation from his family (often around age 10–11), special camps can be particularly helpful. Children with many physical disorders can, of course, enjoy and profit from attending a well-run conventional camp. But if their medical needs are complex or if they are having marked difficulties in coming to terms with their afflictions, a camp for children with their special disorder can be especially helpful. Camps for children with diabetes have existed for over 40 years; more recently, camps for children with other complex disorders, such as hemophilia and cystic fibrosis, have been developed. These camps have been staffed by carefully trained personnel and have medical care promptly available. They offer not only facilities for and supervision of the child's medical regimen but also education for the child (and his family) concerning his disorder and its management.* Just as important, they offer the child an opportunity to share his problems with a group of peers, and to observe the ways in which they cope with problems of their own.

It is also immensely encouraging for your child to learn about public figures — in government, the performing arts, and sports, for ex-

---

*Naturally, it is essential to make sure that the camp follows the same medical regimen that has been prescribed for your child.

ample — who had or have the same disorder he has, and who have, none-theless, made distinguished contributions to society. For example, it was a source of great interest to many asthmatic children who followed the Olympic Games in the summer of 1972 to learn that a long-distance run-ner and a competition swimmer suffered from asthma. Such outstand-ing persons are models the child can strive to be like, at first in his day-dreams, later, perhaps in reality.

Identifying His Assets. The degree to which a child's peers value him is influenced by the manner in which he presents himself to them — especially the degree to which they sense that he accepts and values himself — and by his contributions to the group. Therefore, a major way to help your child cope with the challenge of being physically different is to help him develop personal characteristics, skills, and talents that make a positive contribution to group experience.

Release of Feeling. Although there are many ways you can help your child cope with being different from others, his condition is a troubling fact of his life. He will need opportunities to release his feelings of distress, just as you do, too.

If his condition has developed recently, he will react to the changes within himself. It is almost as though he mourns for his partly ruined body, experiencing many of the characteristic grief reactions you your-self have had (Chapter 1). There may at first be disbelief, followed much later by acknowledgment of the illness, with understandable sadness, resentment, apprehension, and perhaps some feelings of unworthiness and guilt. Even if the disorder is long-standing, changing circumstances will arouse such feelings again and again.

Usually less able than the preschooler to discharge his feelings through his play, the youngster will need frequent opportunities to con-fide in a trusted relative or friend, or perhaps someone a little more detached, such as a favorite teacher, a minister, or a social worker. He will need opportunities to discharge feelings through aggressive but acceptable bodily movement (hitting a punching bag, kicking a ball, or walloping it with a bat). He might be encouraged to pour out his emotions creatively — on a musical instrument, with paint or clay, in story writing or poetry.

The Sense of Accomplishment

A child's self-esteem can be a wellspring of inner contentment in the present as well as a major determinant of his adjustment in adulthood. It has been found among persons with hemophilia, for example, that the young man's view of himself as a socially competent and productive individual is just as significant as the severity of his physical illness, perhaps even more so.

In mid-childhood, a youngster's self esteem is molded by the attitudes and judgments of peers and significant adults as well as by family members. It is influenced significantly by his experiences of accomplishment.

The child's maturation has provided him with a growing capacity to learn, plan, build, and share, as well as the capacity to develop new physical skills. There are at least four major areas in which he can, with appropriate help, experience a sense of accomplishment.

Behavioral Mastery

By mid-childhood, the youngster should have become capable of regulating his instincts and impulses (to hit, grab, smash, smear, for example) so as to conform reasonably well to the standards of his family and his school.* To accomplish such self-mastery, the youngster will need considerable help from his parents. He will need clear and consistent guidelines — family rules — to help him to know what behavior is expected and what is unacceptable. At times, family expectations will need to be reinforced by discipline, such as reprimands or withdrawal of privileges.

Although an occasional slap is no disaster, physical punishment is generally not helpful, and for two major reasons. First, the goal of discipline is to help the child regulate his impulses, his inner tensions and excitements. Physical punishment — spanking, beating, strapping — usually intensifies the child's tension and excitement by stimulating strong emotions such as fear and resentment. A vicious cycle is readily set up — the more the child misbehaves, the more he is spanked, the more excited he feels, the more he misbehaves. Second, it is the responsibility of parents to serve as models, that is to offer the child examples of acceptable ways of expressing aggressive impulses and angry feelings. A parent who hits and spanks is showing the child that his own way of dealing with anger is by physical violence. Can he then justifiably ask the child to do otherwise?

A child needs to be shown channels through which it *is* acceptable to release tension, excitement, and emotions such as anger, resentment,

---

*Impulse control is a major task of development that begins in infancy. It is a task requiring parental help in the form of clear setting of limits, firmness, tact, and patience. It is a task parents of ill children are likely to have difficulty with, as shown in Chapter 3.

and jealousy. Parents need to ask themselves the question, "In what way do I believe it is all right for my child to express his feelings?" Acceptable outlets — talking it over, physical discharge, play equipment — then need to be provided.

In each family, there is a child-rearing value system. It may vary from authoritarianism, in which rules are rigidly reinforced and no questioning by the child is tolerated, to "democracy," in which the wishes of the children are given as much consideration as the parents' — or more. The latter extreme can make children anxious, because they lack the guidelines to reinforce their own still insecure controls. The former extreme deprives the child of experience in decision making and developing confidence in his own judgments. Children need both clear guidelines and opportunities to make judgments and decisions that their parents can accept.

All children test the restrictions imposed on their behavior. Unless they find that the restrictions are consistent and secure, they may learn to manipulate and tyrannize their families in ways that leave all the members, including the child, resentful and anxious. Children at the onset of an acquired illness such as rheumatic fever, for example, may become miserably worried by unusual parental permissiveness, since it suggests that the child must indeed be damaged. Children with long-standing physical disorders sometimes use symptoms to control their families, although usually without full awareness of so doing. For example, a child with lung disease might have violent coughing fits when his wishes were opposed, thus frightening his parents into (resentful) capitulation. (Emotional states do affect the production of secretions in the air passages and do contribute to spasm in the airways.)

For a variety of reasons that have been discussed (in Chapter 3), parents of children with physical disorders can have especial difficulty in setting limits. If a school-age child is allowed to develop a pattern of tyrannizing his family, whether by manifesting frightening behavior or frightening symptoms, attacks or seizures of his illness, professional help is clearly needed. No child whose behavior frequently arouses anger and resentment in those around — reactions he readily senses — can develop a secure sense of accomplishment and personal worth.

Scholastic Accomplishment

School is the major locus of accomplishment in mid-childhood, and parents of children with physical disorders can take steps to increase the likelihood that the school experience is rewarding.

First, parents can strive to insure that the school staff members have realistic expectations concerning the child (page 99). Very few chronic or extended illnesses are associated with brain damage or mental retardation or exert any direct influence on the child's intellectual capabilities. Children with such disorders as asthma, cystic fibrosis, diabetes, hemophilia, leukemia, and kidney disease, for example, may be bright, average, or slow learners, just as may physically healthy children.

Second, parents can collaborate with the school staff in planning for special academic needs (for example, tutorial assistance when illness causes absences) and in dealing with special physical needs. If a teacher seems inappropriately indulgent or apprehensive about a child with a physical disorder, parents may bring this to the attention of someone in a position to discuss it with the teacher — the principal, school social worker, psychologist, guidance counselor, public health nurse.

Learning Problems.   Considerable mental energy is available to the healthy child to direct toward formal learning in school. Hopefully, the child can attain a middle ground between a frantic striving to excel at one extreme and a dread of facing new challenges at the other.

Learning problems may arise from many different sources. They may result from intellectual impairment or from disturbed function of the central nervous system. They may arise from anxiety related to troubled family relationships or from difficulties in controlling aggressive impulses or bodily tensions. They may reflect psychological depression, which is marked by feelings of worthlessness, helplessness, and hopelessness as well as a slowing of mental functions. They may reflect ineffective teaching methods or chaos in the classroom. Since physically healthy children, as well as children with physical disorders, are subject to such problems, should your child develop a learning problem, it must not be quickly concluded that it is caused by his illness. Rather, his problem deserves as careful and thorough an evaluation by medical, educational, and mental health professionals as that of any child.

School Avoidance.   Children commonly express emotional distress through bodily symptoms. A usually healthy child, needing to avoid school, will rarely say that he is afraid to go to school (in fact, he may not even recognize his own fear). Rather, he is likely to complain of a headache or an upset stomach — which, at that moment, he genuinely feels. When such complaints are repeated, especially in the early morning, an observant parent usually suspects a problem connected with school.

It may be more difficult for parents of children with physical disorders to judge such a case. Some such parents do notice that, when their children are faced with an ordinary stress in school, a test, for example, their children's chronic symptoms, such as coughing, wheezing, abdominal cramping and pain, become more severe. (Occasionally, a child indicates his own awareness of this. John, a nine-year-old with asthma, would occasionally announce to his mother in the evening that he probably would not feel well enough for school the next day. The following day, he would invariably waken with a stomachache.) Furthermore, worry or emotional tension may lower the child's tolerance of his usual symptoms. On the other hand, the severity of many physical disorders does characteristically fluctuate. At certain times, the child *is* more severely ill. Therefore, it is extremely difficult for parents to know whether the wiser and kinder course is to urge the child to attend school in spite of his complaints or to encourage him to stay home. A first, prompt step toward a decision is a review of his physical status with his physician, followed by a review of his school experience with his teacher.

A recurrent or prolonged wish to avoid school in a child who is not acutely ill usually indicates emotional distress. In the child up to about third-grade level, it may reflect anxiety about separation from the family. A child with a physical disorder may have had especial difficulty in achieving an adequate sense of independence by school age (see Chapter 4). He may also sense his parents' apprehension about having him move beyond their direct supervision and care. His avoidance of school may represent his behavioral compliance with their unspoken wish to keep him close.

In the slightly older child, school avoidance may also reflect social anxiety — especially fear of rejection by his peers — or a fear of academic failure. It may reflect worry about changes or problems in family life. It may be a response to his parents' wish to shield him from distressing experiences. For example, the parents of a 10-year-old girl with leukemia encouraged her to stay home from school even during periods of symptom-free remission, because of their fear that she would hear from a classmate the name of her illness, which they had tried to conceal from her. In actuality, she had already overheard her father discussing the diagnosis on the telephone.

If school avoidance in a child who is physically able to attend is frequent or prolonged, he is deprived of appropriate contact with his peers, as well as of the learning opportunities that are a major source of his sense of accomplishment. His use of time becomes unstructured. Too readily, in fact, each day becomes a void increasingly filled with rumination about himself, and with despair. The parent who feels pessimistic about the child's expected lifespan (and wonders, "What use is school without a future?") should remember that the quality of the child's present existence is of crucial significance. Goal-directed activity — even completing a school assignment — keeps alive the sense of hope that is the antidote to despair.

It has been found that the more prolonged the period of school avoidance, the more apprehensive the child is on contemplating return. His apprehension may reach the intensity of panic; school avoidance can legitimately be considered a psychological emergency. The close and prompt collaboration of the child's parents, physician, and educational and mental health professionals is often needed to resolve the problem.

Physical Accomplishments and Sports

In our society, it is expected that the boy approaching puberty test and prove his manhood in the arena of physical combat. (As a rule, this expectation does not apply to girls. To the contrary, school-age girls are often supplied with woefully inadequate physical education programs and facilities.) Currently, the sports most emphasized tend to be highly competitive ones — baseball, basketball, and football. Unfortunately, rather than offering experiences in team cooperation and comradeship, such sports emphasize winning — the final score becomes more important than how the game is played. Too often, this attitude is reinforced by physical education teachers and coaches, who derive their own sense of accomplishment from their teams' trophies.

Even healthy youngsters who are awkward, poorly coordinated, or slow runners can experience much misery in sports contests. So may the youngster with a physical disorder that produces faintness, weakness, breathlessness, coughing, and wheezing, or that carries the risk of bleeding or fracture. In addition to his own disability, this youngster may have to deal with the apprehension and sometimes excessive restrictions of his parents. The parents, understandably, worry that the child's activity might result in a worsening of his condition that would disrupt family life and cause physical misery for the child. Unfortunately, however, undue protectiveness usually brings emotional misery to the child and, indirectly, to his family as well.

One of the most agonizing dilemmas faced by parents is whether to safeguard the child's physical existence by every possible means or to give priority to the quality of life even if to do so involves some physical risk. Responsibility for making decisions about physical activity should be shared by parents and the child's physician. Furthermore, medical guidelines are needed concerning the nature and intensity of activity that the child can tolerate. Some can tolerate short bursts of intense activity, as in ice hockey; others can tolerate sustained activity of a milder sort, as in hiking.

Within the doctor's guidelines, parents and teachers can, with some effort and imagination, encourage the child to develop skills in a range of activities that are within his physical capabilities. Such a program might include swimming, fishing, hiking, biking, golf, tennis, badminton, gymnastics, dancing, ice skating, informal softball games, touch football, wrestling, judo, karate. Such activities may require supervision, to determine, for example, that ice skating does not become a forbidden hockey contest or that touch football does not turn into tackle.

Parents can make the environment conducive to sports activities (and attractive to the child's peers also), either on their own private property or in cooperation with neighbors or landlords. Badminton, volleyball, ringtoss, archery, croquet, shooting baskets, Ping-Pong, shuffleboard (on a driveway) are games that can be provided for at reasonable cost in or near the home. Billiards and pool are appealing, and chess has attained status as a "sport" of the mind.

For children with severe disabilities, it is worthwhile exploring community resources. A local Y or rehabilitation center may either offer special facilities or be persuaded to develop such a program. Skill at a sport offers the child not only some contact with his peers and status among them but also a valuable channel through which he can discharge the tension and anger aroused by the frustration of his illness.

The child can participate vicariously in dangerous or forbidden sports (tackle football, ice hockey, horse or car racing) through books, magazines, and television. He can also achieve a certain status by becoming an authority on a sport, its rules and its players. He might prove valuable as a team manager or coach. He can vicariously own a team by developing skill at trading baseball or football cards. He can daydream — the solace available to all human beings who feel frustration at the difference between what they are and what they might wish to be.

Creative Accomplishments

Even if a youngster cannot be physically "worthy" of the gang, as Jonathan lamented (page 96), he can be helped to develop his own unique characteristics and some skills through which he could make a valued contribution to the group. For example, one frail, skinny, poorly coordinated boy became the center of an enthusiastic group of young would-be playwrights because of his interest and talent in dramatics. (The group included some of the most rugged baseball heroes in his class.) In such a fashion, a talent and enthusiasm for story writing, a musical instrument, singing, drawing, or baking, or a well-developed sense of humor, especially if expressed in clever joke telling or cartooning — any such skills can win interest and approval from a child's peers. Furthermore, even those talents that may not necessarily become a center of group activity — painting, weaving, ceramics, stitchery, for example, offer the child valuable ways to express his inner experience and his emotions. Guidance in helping your child identify and develop such talents should be available from the school staff, community centers such as the Y's, Scout leaders, camp counselors, and rehabilitation centers.

Some such activities may develop into lifelong hobbies. For example, a child encouraged to develop an interest in radio may in time become a ham operator. Especially valuable if this young person is restricted and isolated by physical disability, such a skill would enable him to become part of a wide network of human communication.

Household Responsibility

As a society becomes more affluent, opportunities for the individual to attain a sense of significance may be reduced. As the home becomes more affluent, homemaking tends increasingly to become a matter of organizing and integrating. The actual tasks are performed by mechanical instruments, and energy is supplied by electricity. Therefore, fewer and fewer tasks remain that are interesting to and appropriate for the school-age child. In addition, speed has become a goal in itself; parents can almost invariably carry out tasks more swiftly and efficiently than can their offspring.

Furthermore, many of today's parents have achieved their affluent status through intense striving, and retain vivid memories of childhood hardships. They view it as an accomplishment and a privilege to spare their own children any hard work.

For such reasons, many children today lack any significant role in carrying out the tasks of family life. And the child with a physical disorder may be especially deprived in this way because of his parents' wish to make his life as easy and comfortable as possible. Ironically, he may be just the child who most needs a sense of accomplishment in any area available.

Chores assigned to a school-age child need to be selected thoughtfully so that success is attainable; nothing is gained if the jobs are so distasteful that the child habitually forgets or avoids them and the parent is compelled habitually to nag.

Chores can be isolating or sociable. Most children (as well as most homemakers) dislike the isolating ones. Almost any child sent to pick up his room by himself will show remarkable talents for stalling or for evading the task. That same child may cheerfully clean out the garage with his father or fold laundry with his mother: such work can be done sociably and cooperatively, with meaningful communications of thoughts and feelings often taking place.

The child should be assigned only those chores that he has the skills to accomplish competently. It deprives him of satisfaction if, for example, he vacuums a room and then sees his mother redoing it later because he did not meet her standards of thoroughness.

Chores should be time limited. It should be possible to see concrete results within a reasonably short period of time. If the task is one requiring many hours for completion, it is helpful to agree in advance how long the child will work at it, and then perhaps to use a timer or alarm clock to guarantee that the agreement is honored. If concrete results are not especially evident, many children enjoy the visible recognition of a prominently displayed chart on which their accomplishment is recorded.

Chores should be essential tasks. Children are quick to sense the phoniness of made-work. Even if much of the household work is done by electrical appliances, there are still tasks that require human judgments. The child might make out the grocery list or plan a week's menus.

Chores are especially rewarding if they offer the child opportunities for decision making and creativity. One mother snorted, "Big deal!" when it was suggested that her daughter set the dinner table each evening. This mother's idea of table setting was the common but sterile notion of placing a knife, fork, spoon, glass, and paper napkin on a plastic table top. Whoever set her table would learn nothing of creating an appealing environment for the evening meal (almost the only time the family assembled together). She overlooked the attractiveness of brightly colored placemats and tablecloths (today's marvelously patterned, drip-dry sheets make inexpensive cloths), of an interesting centerpiece (composed, perhaps, of driftwood, pine cones, sea shells, or plants), of the charm and warm intimacy of candlelight.

Chores can offer avenues for release of tension. A child can delight in a glorious mess of soapsuds and streams of water to wash the car on a warm day. He can squeeze and pound and slap furiously at a glob of cookie dough, then cook it, with delectable results.

Chore assignment necessitates thoughtful planning as well as consistent supervision. If a parent fails to make clear his expectation that the chore will be completed (and after its completion fails to offer recognition and appreciation), he is subtly letting the child know that he does not value the child's contribution to the household very highly.

Explaining the Illness

Why Tell Him?

Parents find it difficult enough to think about their child's disorder, let alone to have to talk with him about it. Parents often wish the child could be spared any knowledge of his affliction, and they certainly wish him not to dwell on it. They fear that talking about it may increase his tendency to do so, but, in fact, the opposite is usually the case.

The child learns about his disorder in a variety of ways. He may look different, he may have disagreeable symptoms, he may feel tired or sick. At the onset of his illness, there were probably marked changes in the mood and behavior of his family (Chapters 1 and 2) and in their responses to him. Whether recent or longstanding, his illness will have necessitated visits to doctors and perhaps hospitalization. The child will probably have overheard (and only partly understood) conversations among medical people, relatives, and friends. It is inevitable that the child will know there is something wrong with him. Parents acknowledge their awareness of this in the common statement, "He probably knows more than we realize."

The conspiracy of secrecy with which the family of the ill child may surround him (in an effort to spare him knowledge and worry), is the very thing that has been found, again and again, to be the most terrifying to the child. Without realistic knowledge, forced to construct theories in his imagination (that are apt to be more frightening than reality), his fears have no boundaries and he feels utterly alone.

Giving the child some appropriate information can help to reduce his anxiety. Knowing is a way of feeling in charge. It offers a basis for planning how to solve problems. It enables the ill child to make judgments that gradually help him toward independence in managing his medical needs. Knowing helps the child meet the challenge of revealing his needs and problems to his peers. It helps to immunize him against feeling suddenly overwhelmed by their statements or questions. Being told allows the child to communicate with his parents about the illness and prevents him from feeling utterly alone.

How to Explain

Preparing Yourself. From the time he reaches school-age, communicating with your child about his disorder is a fact of daily life; it is not a happening, but a continuous, ever-changing, sometimes painful, often rewarding experience. Whether the disorder has been present since birth, or whether it was acquired later, your school-age child's developing intellectual capacities increasingly enable him to use information constructively in coping with his disorder.

If you prepare yourself for this responsibility, it is likely that your own feelings of helplessness about your child will be reduced, you will feel less dread about dealing with his questions, and you will be able to create a climate in which your child is free to inquire. Your attitudes about communication, readily sensed by your child, will be just as important as the information you give him.

Since one can't explain what he himself does not understand, your first task is to inform yourself (Chapter 8). You will need repeated opportunities to review your knowledge of the illness and to ask new questions.

It may also be helpful to rehearse in your thoughts what you might say to your child if he asked some of the significant questions discussed in this chapter. You might rehearse your explanations by putting them into words with a trusted relative or friend or with other parents of children with the same affliction.

Defusing the Communication. Although a release of feeling in moderate doses may be helpful to your child and to you, a dramatic loss of control would distress both of you. Therefore, it is often useful to discuss your child's disorder with him in a situation in which the intensity of the communications can be reduced through activity. Taking a walk with him, mixing cookie dough, making beds, raking leaves — any such ordinary activities allow both of you to be as casual as you need, to release tension through movement, and to avoid too much emotion-laden eye-to-eye gazing.

Sometimes it is easier to talk about difficult topics through an intermediary. School-age children can still talk through puppets, listen to or tell a story about a make-believe child with the same disorders, or discuss a popular figure, perhaps a well-known ballplayer, runner, or swimmer who has the same affliction. The latter approach can be especially helpful if your child has never asked direct questions: "I was reading about so-and-so in the Olympic Games. It said that he has had a health condition like yours."

Clarifying His Questions. An 11-year-old boy with mild asthma constructed a series of riddles for his mother one rainy afternoon. The first on the list was: "How does childhood end and how does death begin?" "Oh God," wondered his mother silently, "where do I even begin with this one?" Exclaiming, "Wow, that's a hard one," she noticed her son's face was puckered in a mischievous grin. "It's really a very simple one, Mom," he reassured. With good fortune, knowing his current interest in word structure and crossword puzzles, she guessed, "With the letter *D*." "Correct!" "Whew!" his mother felt inwardly, but at the same time stored away for future reflection a question as to whether he was experiencing some unacknowledged worry about his condition.

Overwhelming a child with too much information is no more useful than withholding needed facts. Most children need to have periods when they can keep from themselves — through denial — an awareness of the chronicity or seriousness of their condition. Try to understand what your child is actually asking at the particular time. One of several simple comments might be helpful: "I'll tell you what I understand about that, Bill, but first tell me what you've heard (or read) about it — how do you suppose it works." Or, "I'll try to answer your question, Laura, but I wonder what made you think of it?"

Such strategy serves several purposes. If your child's question arises from thoughts and imaginings more frightening than the reality, it enables him to reveal his worries and you to give reassurance. For example, the same boy with asthma one day thus revealed his sense of panic. Half listening to a TV commercial for a bronchodilator, he understood the frenetic announcer to say, "Nine out of 10 people who have an attack don't make it!" Even though the boy's condition was mild, he understood this as a prediction that he would almost certainly die during a wheezing spell. Fortunately, he confided this terrifying thought to his mother, who reassured him immediately and also arranged for the boy to have a reassuring consultation with his doctor.

Clarifying the basis for your child's questions also enables you to stay attuned to his ever-changing ideas (which are influenced by his intellectual development, as well as by how he feels, what he reads or hears, and his medical care), and to evaluate how clearly he has understood information given in the past.

Permitting Release of Feeling.   On occasion, when your child asks a question, he may be seeking an opportunity to release his feelings rather than looking for information. The tone of voice in which he asks and his facial expression may give you clues to this. If, in exasperation, he asks, "*Why* do I start coughing every time I try to shoot baskets?", it can be more helpful to respond to his feelings than to give an explanation about bronchospasm or mucus in the airways. "That's rough, Paul. It must make you mad and discouraged that it happens." Knowing that you understand his feelings is comforting to him. Hearing you put them into words offers him a helpful example of using words to express emotion, and if he does this himself, the intensity of his feelings may be much reduced.

The opportunity to release his feelings may be all that he is seeking at that moment. If, however, he is asking for more information, he should then be better able to assimilate it. Apprehension, anger, sorrow, or guilt can interfere with a child's capacity to listen and to understand, just as it does with an adult's.

If your child has opportunity to release feeling frequently and in small doses, it is almost as though he becomes immunized against a buildup and an explosion of emotion that could be overwhelming to him and to you. Furthermore, a surprising number of children can begin to use irony or frank humor as an acceptable way of discharging excitement, shame, apprehension, or anger. For example, an eight-year-old boy with cystic fibrosis would say wryly, "When God made me, he didn't do a very good job. Couldn't we send in for some spare parts?" A number of boys with the same disorder have dealt with the embarrassment of their flatulence by making jokes about it.

What to Explain

Information about his illness can be useful to a child only if it is given in terms he can understand. School-age children have a rapidly growing capacity to think in ways adults consider reasonable or logical. They increasingly understand the relationships of objects, persons, or experiences — relationships of size and color, relationships of position in space, relationships of cause and effect, for example.

They increasingly understand that certain properties of a substance may remain unchanged even while some of its characteristics vary. For example, the same quantity of juice will appear different in a tall thin glass than when in a short, fat glass. Medicine may have the form of a liquid or of a pill but still have the same effect on the body. At the same time, the child is grasping that under some conditions substances are transformed into quite different matter. For example, they begin to understand that food is transformed into other substances that the body uses and that the unused portions are eliminated as wastes.

Around nine years of age, many children show a marked increase in knowledge about the structures and functions of their bodies. Their ideas are becoming similar to those of adults. However, until children are about 11 or 12 years old, their ideas are based primarily on personal observation and experience. Their ideas about the abstract are still vague. Children guess, for example, that the liver, which they cannot see or feel, is "so you can live." Although they understand that the body uses food, they have little understanding of what *energy* actually is other than the way they feel when they are "peppy" or "energetic."

Similarly, children's notions about their health conditions are related to their own direct experience and observation. Among a group of diabetic children in a special study, the majority of six- and seven-year-olds realized that when urine was tested with Clinitest, the development of the orange-red color (which they had actually observed) meant that a large amount of sugar was present in the urine. However, only among the group six years older, the 12- and 13-year-olds, did the majority grasp such crucial but abstract information about their disease as the fact that blood sugar is increased in uncontrolled diabetes or that insulin causes blood sugar to decrease.

Children with cystic fibrosis explained their illness in terms of what they had directly experienced. They referred either to mucus (or "phlegm," "stuff," "junk," "crap") in the chest or to bowel problems. "The chest gets all clogged up with mucus and that makes you cough." "The mucus in your chest clogs up your lungs and makes you cough a lot, and it does something to your breathing — makes you wheezy." "My bowels ain't working right, so it comes out stinky."

A few children in this group were unable to give any explanation of their condition although they communicated anxiety about it. "I've got trouble inside me." "I don't know [what cystic fibrosis is], but it's not good to have."

What a child in mid-childhood can grasp about his condition is influenced by several factors: (1) his general understanding of bodily processes, including information gleaned from school biology courses, misinformation gathered from his playmates, tantalizing "secrets" glimpsed in the neighbor's copy of *Playboy*, (2) the family attitudes about curiosity (is it acceptable or is it "not nice" to wonder and ask about bodily functions?), (3) family attitudes about discussing his disorder (when he tries to talk about it, does a tense body and worried look on his parent's face communicate, "Please don't ask"?), (4) the intensity of his worry about himself (an apprehensive child can misunderstand or block out realistic information just as readily as an adult), (5) his intellectual capabilities (whether he is quick, average, or slow in grasping new ideas), and (6) the actual information given. Basically, however, the youngster can be expected to grasp only the information that is related to bodily functions he feels or observes.

It is difficult for parents, as well as for many health professionals, to explain a complex illness in terms a child can understand. Help may be sought from written materials prepared for children by some of the voluntary health agencies, as well as from your child's science, biology, or health teacher. Such a teacher may be able to help you interpret medical information in terms of bodily processes the child could be expected to understand.

From time to time, it is useful to review with your child his ideas about his illness. This helps you judge whether your explanations have been meaningful. One way of doing this is, in a relaxed moment, to wonder, "John, if you were going to explain diabetes to another kid who had just learned he had it, what would you tell him?"

What's It Called?   When a child has a potentially life-threatening disorder, some parents go to great lengths to conceal its name from the child. They fear, understandably, that if the child should connect the name *cystic fibrosis* or *leukemia* with himself, he would then become aware that he is in danger. He might see a fund-raising appeal on TV, in which the most heartbreaking aspects of the illness may be emphasized to persuade the public to give generously. He may read in the newspapers or in books — in biographies of sports heroes, for example — of others who died from his disease.

Such exposures may — and do — occur, and the child will then indeed need a trusted person in whom to confide his fears. Unfortunately, trying to keep the name of his disorder a secret rarely (if ever) protects the child from awareness of his danger. His family and their friends are likely to mention the disorder by name within his earshot; his doctors and nurses will discuss his disorder by name — in fact, he may regularly attend a cystic fibrosis clinic, for example. His diagnosis will be written on requisitions for laboratory studies or x-rays and in his medical record. There may be pamphlets about the disorder in his household. A relative may have been afflicted with the same illness. Difficult as it is for parents to accept, there is probably no way short of keeping him isolated in a soundproof room to prevent a school-age child from learning the name of his disorder. And it is the attempts to maintain secrecy, and leaving the child in isolation with his suspicions and fears, that overwhelm him most grievously. Telling the child the name of his disorder is not — as parents fear — the same as telling him he is going to die.

Why Me?   "It's not really something bad," declared an eight-year-old boy with kidney disease. "You can't help it." An eleven-and-a-half-year-old with a heart defect explained, "I was born with it — it ain't my fault." Both boys revealed a major concern of ill children from the preschool years (see page 67) through adolescence, "Am I to blame for being sick?" This is such a troubling, common, and recurring concern of children that it is worthwhile to reassure your child about it occasionally, whether or not he directly asks. Even if the cause of the disorder is not entirely understood, as in nephrosis or leukemia, for example, one can say, "The doctors don't know exactly what starts this off, but they do know that it isn't because of anything children do, or even think of doing, to themselves!"

When an illness is inherited, parents are apt to feel responsible and extremely regretful, perhaps even quite guilty. Therefore, it is very difficult to explain to their child that the disorder was passed from parent to child. It may seem like confessing, "I did this to you." The parent may fear that the child will then blame him (and this does occasionally happen. When a child is angry at a parent, he is apt to use as ammunition any thought that pops into his mind). It is often more comfortable — and realistic — to explain, "This is a condition that runs in our family." You can point out that all families have certain physical characteristics that please them — perhaps a tendency to be tall or to have jet-black hair — and certain characteristics that displease them — nearsightedness, for example. Some traits that run in a family cause illness. You might point out that although you feel very sorry that it is this way, the trait came to you from your parents, and to them from their parents, and it is not anyone's fault at all. There are no perfect human beings. (Generally, it is not until the teen years that youngsters can sufficiently well comprehend the abstract mysteries of genetics to begin to deal meaningfully with the difficult possibility of passing the illness on to their own children.)

Children, as well as their parents, search for an explanation for their illness that gives it some kind of meaning. Sometimes a sensitive clergyman can help a child find meaning in his illness. Often, however, it is the parent who must support the child in enduring the difficulty of not knowing why this happened to him. Just allowing him to talk about it, and acknowledging, "We don't understand why such things happen, and it's awfully hard not to know," offers some comfort.

Will I Always Have It?   "Mommy, there is a lot the doctors don't know about this, and it's going to take a long time," gravely declared a six-and-a-half-year-old girl with kidney disease, when her mother fretted, "Tell the doctors to hurry and make you well." In such a manner, even a young school-age child can show some realistic awareness of the chronicity of certain disorders.

However, children can usually accept a chronic problem only little by little, over a prolonged period. They need — and have a right — to be sustained by hope, just as you do. Therefore, to tell a child that he will have his problem "forever" or "all your life" may leave him feeling discouraged, hopeless, even overwhelmed. It may be more encouraging — and still be realistic — to say, "Right now, the doctors can do a lot to help you feel better, but they don't yet know how to get rid of the illness. We will have to manage with it for a while, and it may be quite a long while. But doctors all over the world are studying this problem, and they are learning more about this sickness all the time. We can certainly hope that one day they will know how to make children like you completely healthy again."

The Dreaded Question

"Mommy, am I going to die?" Can there be a question more dreaded by parents? Devoted parents of the healthiest child find that such a question stirs deep sadness, even though they may confidently say, "Not for a long, long time." For parents of an ill child, the question is a painful shaft penetrating to their deepest fears. Inwardly and silently they may long to shout, "Oh, Jill, don't make me think of that. Don't ask it, don't ask it." But the question, whether spoken or unspoken, is inevitable.

In other times and other lands, where the usual lifespan has been short, where large families and tribes live close together, where epidemics often rage, children are faced with death in personal, daily experience. In our own society, even though the topic of death is often avoided like a shameful secret, or an appalling failure of our technology, any child who reads or watches television is confronted, sometimes brutally, with images of death in its most violent manifestations — in war, assassination, riot, tornado, and plane crash.

Children with health problems witness fund-raising appeals and commercial advertisements on TV that often emphasize the dangerous aspects of disease. They readily (and sometimes quite incorrectly) relate these to themselves. Children with health problems are sometimes confronted brutally with questions from their classmates — "I heard my mom tell my dad that you're probably going to be dead by next year. Is that true?" An angry or frightened brother or sister may make fearful predictions — one little girl would "win" fights with her ill brother by declaring, "You're going to be with the angels pretty soon — so there!"

Children who attend specialty clinics in a hospital may notice that another patient, who used to be there every month, has mysteriously disappeared. Children who have had a relative who has died from the same disorder — or a disorder the child imagines to be the same — worry about the same fate's befalling them.

What Meaning Has Death?   Between six and eight years of age, the child gradually leaves behind his earlier beliefs that death is temporary, only partial, and much like sleep (Chapter 4). He may now imagine it as an external force, somewhat human and often masculine in form (the Grim Reaper of folklore) that carries people away. This concept is probably a significant factor in the nighttime fears, fantasies, and bad dreams that are common at this age.

Around nine or 10 years of age, many children begin to grasp the idea of death as the universal and permanent end of bodily life. The body after death is no longer imagined to be existing somewhere else (as the preschooler thinks) but as withering away and turning to dust like the dried petals of a flower.

Although the child can grasp this idea intellectually, the idea of not-being is an affront to his sense of self (as it is to all of us). Furthermore, the idea of death is apt to remain associated in his mind with angry feelings, with thoughts of pain, and with the sadness of separation. Therefore, he will tend to avoid and deny the likelihood of such a thing's happening to him.

Religious beliefs, especially belief in an afterlife and the thought of reunion with the beloved family, can offer comfort in some instances. Even if his own family does not hold such beliefs, a school-age child becomes aware that others do. Many parents who do not have a personal religious faith feel comfortable in acknowledging, "Yes, many people do believe in that. We feel that we don't know for sure whether it is true or not." Comforting to some, belief in an afterlife can also be a source of terror to a child who is convinced that he is bad or unworthy and who expects punishment after death by an angry God.

Helpful Measures.   There is no way it can be made easy for you to answer your child's questions about his own death. They will inevitably arouse sadness, fear, and perhaps some guilt deep inside you. Your first task may have to be to acknowledge your feeling, since your child will surely sense it from your facial expression, tone of voice, and from your movements (you may tense up or quickly turn away): "Gosh, Jennifer, what a sad thought that is. It just isn't easy for any of us to talk about dying!"

It is most helpful to explore what prompted the child's question at this moment. If the child's medical status is reasonably good, you might say, "You're getting on very well, Stevie. I wonder what made you think of dying just now?" This may encourage your child to tell you about a frightening experience or comment he has heard. He may have learned from the newspapers or TV of the death of others with his illness. He may have learned of the death of a child he knew in the hospital, or have been reminded of a relative with the same illness.

If he tells you he has heard that others have died from his illness, you will need to acknowledge, "Yes, it's true, that has happened." You can then draw on many different sources of reassurance: each case is different — some are diagnosed sooner, some later; some are severe, some mild; some people don't get to the doctor soon enough or often enough; some don't follow his advice.

Parents, desperately wishing to reassure and protect the child, sometimes say, "I'm not going to *let* you die!" Sadly, it is a promise no parent can fulfill. This the parent really knows. And the child, whose increasing realism should be helping him understand that parents don't have magical powers, will come to know it also. However, many parents find they can combine realism and reassurance: "Nobody on earth knows for sure how long they're going to live (some parents add, "That's something God decides"), but I certainly hope and expect that you and I are going to be together for a long time" (can any parent say more?). You can remind him of all that he and you can do together to help him (the treatment program). You can remind him of all that others are doing to help him, and of the research to learn more about his illness and to find better medicines.

During a period of severe illness, a child's question about his own death usually expresses his awareness that he is dangerously ill and represents an appeal for reassurance. He urgently needs the opportunity for communication with a trusted adult who can listen to his thoughts and worries.

Only a rare child can bear to hear, "Yes, you are dying." Only rare parents can bear to tell him this. Some do, particularly those believing in reunion in afterlife (the poignant last words of one boy thus informed by his father were "See you later, Dad").

For the majority of children, it is most helpful to acknowledge the worry, "You must be feeling scared, Paul"; to explain that he is very sick, and that feeling so bad is naturally worrying. It is then important to reassure him that the doctors and nurses do know how to take care of him and that his family will be close at hand.

If Communication Is Unbearable. Parents of school-age children sometimes remark, "He never asks questions about his condition." Such parents usually wish *not* to know what thoughts are in the ill child's mind, imagining that knowing would be unbearable. Their children have sensed their parents' distress, and have gradually learned not to inquire about troubling subjects. Even parents who usually communicate effectively find that at times, especially if the child is dangerously ill, they reach the limit of what they can bear to allow their children to tell them or to ask.

Unfortunately, the burden of illness is much heavier if borne alone. This is true for the sick child and his parent as well. It is therefore essential that each of you has access to trusted and sensitive persons in whom each can confide his thoughts, hopes, and fears.

Managing the Medical Regimen

Understanding the Treatment

People — adults *and* children — feel less helpless and frightened when there is an action they can take to cope with a problem. Therefore, it can increase your child's sense of mastery to realize that by taking medicine, following a diet, doing his therapy, he is taking action to control his illness.

Furthermore, a growing understanding of the purpose of treatment will enable the child to become responsible for a wider range of such actions. For example, he will become able to make significant observations about his bodily functions and sensations (such as episodes of shakiness or faintness, wheezing spells, or change in bowel activity) and report them to his parents and doctor.

However, through the elementary-school years, a child's understanding of his medical regimen develops slowly, and it is easy to overestimate or to underestimate it. By six or seven years of age, boys with hemophilia have been found to understand that bumps or falls might cause internal bleeding and should be reported to their mothers. But many children this age are unready to judge what additional action should be taken. For example, only one half of a group of six- to seven-year-old children with diabetes knew that they should take sugar or juice when they felt shaky or dizzy. In contrast, the majority (85%) of eight- to nine-year-olds understood it.

Boys eight to 11 years old with cystic fibrosis were found to grasp in simple terms the purpose of inhalation therapy and postural drainage. Typical concepts were, "to see if the phlegm will loosen and help you cough it up"; "to get the junk out of your lungs"; "the mucus in your chest clogs up your lungs and can make you cough a lot and do something to your breathing — make you wheezy." Typical concepts concerning the enzymes prescribed to aid digestion included, "to help digest your food and get strength out of your food"; "if you don't take it you'll feel rotten and always be going to the bathroom."

Such concepts, which are fairly realistic, refer to bodily products, functions, or sensations that have been observed or experienced (mucus, coughing, gaining strength, feeling rotten, going to the bathroom). Even the 11-year-olds, regardless of intelligence, had difficulty grasping the more abstract ideas of bodily processes that could not be directly observed or experienced. A typical confusion between fact and fancy is revealed in one youngster's theory (quoted as he stated it): "Cotazym tightens the bowels — usually they're loose and runny because a part of the digestive system is missing. Cotazym sends the enzymes of a pig and a pig usually eats anything. It helps take the place of a part that's missing."

Similarly, in the study of youngsters with diabetes, it was found that not until the early teens was the majority able to understand crucial but abstract ideas such as the fact that blood sugar is elevated in uncontrolled diabetes or that one action of insulin is to lower blood sugar. Thus, most children under 12 or 13 years of age seem poorly equipped to make independent judgments about their treatment needs.

As the child's understanding of treatment grows, he should be helped to develop realistic expectations. That is, he needs to understand whether the treatment is expected to prevent, to control, or to cure episodes of illness. School-age children are increasingly capable of taking actions in the present that will have results in the future (unlike the preschooler, who expects immediate results from his actions). However, if the expected future result does not come about, they readily become discouraged and feel hopeless about treatment. For example, a child with asthma or cystic fibrosis may suppose that his medicine is going to cure his cough, whereas in reality it can only be expected to reduce bronchospasm or loosen secretions. If, after several weeks or months of taking medicine, he continues to have spasms of coughing, it is natural for him to conclude either that the medicine is worthless or that his is a hopeless case.

Your child needs to know whether or not the treatment will be uncomfortable or even painful. If it is, he will be better able to cooperate if he is allowed occasionally to protest and to release his feelings of sadness and resentment about the discomfort.

Your child needs to know whether or not the treatment will cause side effects that might change his appearance or produce unfamiliar sensations in his body. Without such understanding, he may conclude that any side effects are new and alarming symptoms of his illness.

Your child should be told if his need for treatment is likely to increase at certain times, so that an increase won't be interpreted as frightening evidence that he is getting worse. For example, a child with diabetes should be prepared for the fact that if he is injured or has an infectious illness, or even during a period of normal rapid growth, his need for insulin may increase.

Because his sense of safety may be associated with the present treatment, your child will need help in understanding any major changes in his treatment program that result from new medical knowledge. For example, an eight-year-old boy with cystic fibrosis declared that a boy would sleep in a mist tent "to help the mucus in his lungs — to make him breathe. The mucus in his lungs could stop him from breathing." An 11-year-old asserted that a boy would sleep in the tent "to loosen up the phlegm so he can live and not die." Not long after, the medical regimen for these boys was changed, and the use of the mist tent was discontinued. One can imagine how frightened such youngsters would have felt without considerable interpretation and reassurance.

Moving toward Independent Management

Through mid-childhood, the youngster continues his erratic course toward independence. The progress is rarely smooth, more likely occurring in fits and starts. Especially as he approaches puberty, the child characteristically emits contradictory signals: it is as though one hand beckons and the other hand gestures, "Keep away." The message seems to be, "Don't get too close, but don't desert me, either."

Such communications tend to carry over into the medical regimen, and parents often find themselves vacillating between maintaining strict control (which may foster mounting rebellion as the child approaches the teen years) and giving over responsibility to the child too completely. One mother, exasperated by her child's repeated protests about treatment, declared finally, "OK, it's your life, Kenneth. Do it or don't do it — it's up to you." Unfortunately, and understandably, Kenneth interpreted this declaration to mean that his mother didn't care deeply about his well-being — or his life — and he was flooded with feelings of sadness and futility.

Children between seven and 11 years of age are unlikely to be ready to take full responsibility for their home treatment. For example, boys in the study carried out by Dr. Axelrod and the author made it clear that they would submit to inhalation therapy only if someone "made them" or "told them to do it." (A few acknowledged that they would first "try to get out of it.") Their need for supportive adult authority was natural, since they had unavoidable mixed feelings about the therapy. As one 11-year-old put it, a boy would "feel good because it helps clean out your lungs," but "feel bad because you might be right in the middle of a game." Or, as another explained, "A boy would feel embarrassed because the other kids don't have to do it." Even those boys who accepted responsibility for taking their medication tended to expect and need parental reminders.

Some forgetting is natural, since forgetting to take medicine is a way of pushing the illness out of one's thoughts. Furthermore, school-age children, whether healthy or ill, can often save face with their peers if they can declare, "My mother *made* me," when doing something regarded as monstrously undesirable, like wearing boots in the rain or taking a pill.

On the other hand, 8- and 9-year-old boys with hemophilia have been found to derive a significant sense of pride and confidence from cooperating actively in the management of their bleeding crises. It would appear most effective, therefore, for parents to engage their school-age children in a cooperative effort to carry out home treatment, assigning the child as much responsibility as he appears ready to accept, but making it clear that the parent is standing by ready to assist, remind, encourage, or even occasionally say, "I insist that you do it because I care about you."

Reminding readily becomes nagging, which is tiresome for both parent and child. Nagging can often be minimized if impersonal reminders are used. Rules, regulations, and rituals are important for most children in this age group in helping them keep strong impulses in check. The child with a physical disorder may respond positively to the use of a chart or checklist to record his treatments and a schedule to plan them. The parent can thus say, "It's time for your treatment." This may be more acceptable than "You must do your treatment now," which prompts some children to respond, "I won't!"

It is essential that the parent learn from the child's physician whether or not flexibility is permissible and whether the child can have some opportunities for exercising his own judgment and making his own decisions. A group of boys with cystic fibrosis was presented with an imaginary situation in which one boy, Ralph, was at a party and chocolate cake was served. Ralph knew that the cake would cause a stomachache. The boys were asked what they believed Ralph would do. The majority indicated that they thought Ralph would take some "to go along with the crowd," in spite of the discomfort to follow. Some of the problems were summed up by one boy: "He might feel disgusted because he'd like to eat like the rest of his friends, and have a big helping so it looked like he really enjoyed the party. . . . It also gets to be embarrassing because people don't ask you all the time exactly how much you want, and they cut a chunk off and hand it to you, and here you are with this big chunk, and [you] eat it and get sick or you just eat a little of it and then everybody would be kind of embarrassed [because] when they looked at him his plate's full of chocolate cake still. . . . All his friends would probably have all these big pieces like they'd be part of the crowd and he wished he could eat a lot but then he gets stomachaches."

It is of concern that only two boys thought of anticipating the problem in advance and planning for it by increasing their medicine. To be sure, with some disorders the medical regimen must be strictly followed. In others, however, the child can be allowed some flexibility if he, his doctor, and his parents plan together how special situations like parties could be dealt with.

Special Problems

In a disturbingly large proportion of families including children with health impairments, home treatment is carried out incorrectly, sporadically, or abandoned altogether. Obviously, the child is then endangered physically. Perhaps just as important, child and family are endangered emotionally. The child is likely to conclude that he is considered either hopeless or worthless. And sooner or later, the parents are likely to experience tormenting guilt. A breakdown of the treatment can sometimes be prevented or corrected if several common sources of difficulty are considered.

Bodily Exposure and Contact.   Family attitudes concerning exposure of the body vary. Even in a casual, permissive family, however, bodily privacy becomes increasingly important to children beginning from about eight to 10 years of age. It is likely that this attitude is related to the child's increasing awareness of sexual maturation, whether actual or expected, and the self-consciousness such awareness engenders.* Furthermore, children are increasingly embarrassed by close physical contact with their parents (cuddling, hugging, and kissing).

Some home therapies (for example, injections, physiotherapy,

---

*There is a persistent myth in our society that girls wish to conceal and boys to expose their bodies and bodily functions. This belief is reflected in the design of school bathrooms and locker rooms. In the boys' rooms there may be exposed urinals, open toilet stalls, and a common shower. Such arrangements deny privacy to boys. Many boys, and especially those with physical problems, are caused considerable and unnecessary embarrassment.

postural drainage) require exposure of the body or direct physical contact between child and parent. Parents are perplexed and often annoyed if their children respond with giggling, squirming, silliness, or outright refusals — all signs of the child's self-consciousness.

On the other hand, some parents report that their ill children seem to show an undue interest in physical closeness. Such an interest was reported by two mothers of 11-year-old boys with cystic fibrosis. One of them wondered how to handle her son's request to kiss her on the lips "so I can practice before I start dating." It was suggested that the mother point out that mothers and sons don't kiss like "dates" because their feelings about each other, although affectionate, are quite different from those between dating couples. She was encouraged to ask whether other family members would take over portions of the treatment that involved body-to-body contact so that the boy would not be exposed to so much unsettling physical closeness to his mother.

Most children begin to outgrow their intense physical attachment to and tender feelings toward a parent by the close of early childhood (pages 59-61). Therapies requiring physical manipulations may tend to cause such attachment to persist.

Whether it is child or parent who is made the more uncomfortable by the bodily exposure and contact, embarrassment is likely to lead to avoidance of treatment. It is important to discuss with the doctor and the physiotherapist or inhalation therapist alternate ways of administering treatment. The child might learn to administer some injections himself under supervision. The child might learn to use a mechanical vibrator in place of some of the "clapping" in postural drainage. Even when assistance is needed with the back, the appliance might be more tolerable than the parent's hand. Might someone with a less intense relationship to the child be taught to administer treatment, perhaps a relative or a friend with whom the parent could exchange favors? A group of parents of ill children in the same community might share the fee of a public health nurse or therapist for treatment done at home, and perhaps rotate homes.

Denial or Concealment of the Disorder. A primary concern of school-age children is that their disorder will be revealed to their peers (pages 95-97). Since medical treatment is often a giveaway, children imagine that if they avoid their pill, injection, diet, or therapy, they can avoid disclosure. As has been pointed out, children need support and practical advice in finding ways to talk to friends about their disability and in enduring the temporary embarrassment or avoidance that may follow. Parents also need to exercise tact in deciding when and how the treatment is to be carried out, so that the youngster is not exposed unnecessarily to interruption of group activities or to having an outsider barge in while a procedure is being carried out. A youngster who persistently feels that his treatment makes him an odd-ball might profit greatly from a session in a camp for children with similar disorders.

Carrying out the treatment forces the child (and parent) to acknowledge that he has a medical problem. Many children manage to maintain an intermittent denial of their disorder. That is, except when there is a period of acute illness, they are able to put it out of their thoughts at least some of the time. Such denial is appropriate and can be helpful unless it becomes so pervasive and rigid that the child refuses medical care as unnecessary. Such an attitude often signals that there is intense, underlying anxiety. The child's denial should certainly be discussed with his doctor, and it is most likely that consultation with a mental health professional will be needed.

The Oppositional-Independent Stance.   The treatment program sometimes becomes the battleground on which conflicts between parent and child concerning independence are fought out. The risk of this tends to increase as the child approaches puberty. At the first signs of such a struggle, it is valuable to consider five relevant questions:

First, has the responsibility for the treatment program been genuinely shared by parent and child? Alternately, has the parent either denied the child any active role in carrying out treatment or imposed too much responsibility on him ("It's your life, Kenneth")?

Second, has the parent found out, and informed the child, whether there can be some flexibility in carrying out the treatment program (for example, about eating cake at a birthday party)? If there can, is the child allowed some opportunities to make his own judgments about his actions (perhaps deciding to take a small piece of cake, even knowing he may have a stomachache later).

Third, are there other areas in the child's life in which he has appropriate opportunities for independence in decision making and actions?

Fourth, has conflict been defused by using impersonal aids such as schedules, rules, or charts, rather than by relying on verbal reminders (often viewed as "bugging me" by the child)?

Fifth, has the parent made it clear to the child that the family is committed to the treatment (however disagreeable) because they care deeply about the child's well-being?

Abandoning Treatment.   Some parents capitulate to the child's protests and abandon treatment. This rarely occurs simply because the parent fails to understand the purpose of treatment. It is more likely to occur because the parent can no longer endure the anger, apprehension, sadness, and guilt that the disorder, the treatment, and the child's protests arouse in him. It may occur because the parent can no longer endure thoughts of the illness; by stopping treatment, he desperately attempts to put the illness out of his mind. It may result from a sense of hopelessness, especially if another member of the family has died from the same disorder.

The child may interpret the abandonment of treatment in several ways. He may strive to believe that in some mysterious way his disorder has gone away (but wonder why he still has symptoms). He may suppose that the treatment was worthless. He may imagine that his case is hopeless. Most tragic, he may conclude that his parents no longer care about him.

Breakdown of the treatment program is a medical emergency, psychological as much as physical. All helping resources must be utilized to evaluate what is invariably a complex and crucial problem.

It is an emergency that often develops slowly and insidiously. For this reason, any caring person — teacher, relative, friend, clergyman, social worker — who notices the first signs of a breakdown, forgotten or irregular treatments, has a responsibility to encourage the parents and the child to seek help.

Hospitalization

Sources of Stress

In early childhood, hospitalization subjects the young child to a variety of stresses (Chapter 4), the most significant of which are likely to be separation anxiety and fear of bodily mutilation and pain. In midchildhood, additional worries become prominent. An understanding of their nature can help parents and staff reassure the child effectively.

Fear of Loss of Control.   Although the younger child may be keenly worried about loss of control over bodily functions, as well as about "babyish behavior," he tends to judge himself less harshly than do children of between seven and 11 years of age. For a youngster in midchildhood, receiving intimate bodily care (being bathed, fed, toileted, dressed) tends to arouse contradictory feelings. The care may be welcomed, even enjoyed, when it is most needed, but the child may also feel intense shame because he is accepting care "like a baby." If (even worse), he were to burst into tears or have a temper tantrum, wet his bed or soil his clothes, such a youngster would probably feel very guilty and lose respect for himself. In fact, among hospitalized children 10 years of age or older, the concern about self-mastery is so strong that a central fear is that of being given a drug or anesthetic that would cause the child to lose control.

Fear of Exposure.   As the child begins to look forward to the physical changes of puberty, there is often a heightened wish for bodily privacy. The bodily exposure and manipulations consequent to medical and nursing care may arouse feelings of humiliation and great distress. The distress may be particularly intense if the child is one of the many who imagine that they contributed to their illnesses through some "bad" thought, wish, or action. An eight-year-old girl who had (like most young girls) explored the structure and sensations of her vulva with her fingers and who feared that she might be considered "disgusting" for so doing, became desperately upset when asked to collect a urine specimen. She confessed to her mother her fear that the doctor would be able to look at the specimen and somehow know her guilty secret.

Fear of Social Disadvantage.   School activities constitute a major source of accomplishment in mid-childhood; a sense of kinship with his peers contributes to the child's self-esteem and supports his strivings toward independence. Hospitalization interrupts and interferes with schoolwork and contact with friends. Hospitalized children, therefore, have many realistic worries that they will lose their standing in the group, fall behind in accomplishment, and be unable to compete after discharge. Such worries may become especially prominent as the time for discharge approaches. They are readily overlooked by parents and staff, who may expect the child to rejoice at the prospect of his return to outside life.

Fear of Abandonment.   By mid-childhood, most youngsters are able to cope with periods of separation from their families. They are capable of some realism in understanding the roles of other adults. They can, for example, observe that nurses and doctors have special skills that their parents do not have. When they are feeling sick, they may feel safer to know that their care is supervised by specially trained people, especially if they sense that their parents trust these people to help them.

However, hospital nurses and doctors are busy people and not continuously available. Furthermore, even children who are usually highly independent are likely to feel an intensified need for the comfort and reassurance of their parents' presence when they are ill. One of the deepest fears of children (and of persons of any age) is that of being abandoned to face a frightening or painful ordeal alone.

Fear of Permanent Physical Disability.   The young hospitalized child fears pain and mutilation of his body intensely. In mid-childhood, the youngster's increasing realism, and his capacity to understand the idea of permanence, exposes him to a new dimension of this fear, that of permanent physical disability and of death. The thought of death, of ceasing to be, is such an outrage to the child's sense of self that he is likely to find a variety of ways of denying or avoiding it much of the time. However, the idea of permanent physical disability is likely to be kept quite alive in his thoughts, reinforced frequently by his observations of other children with crutches, casts, bandages, intravenous tubes, heart pacemakers, and oxygen tents. He may readily suppose that his fate is to be similar to theirs, and another child's distress may arouse panic in him.

Reactions to Stress

The responses to stress characteristic of early childhood (pages 84-86) continue to be observed up to the teen years. The child may lose interest in his surroundings and seem withdrawn into himself. He may seem sad, weepy, and apathetic. He may show regression, behaving in more babyish ways than usual. He may react with outbursts of angry or panicky protest, or he may become compliant and docile — too good and too anxious to please. He may, especially if he is approaching puberty, appear stoical, enduring his misery bravely and without even appropriate complaint.

His responses and feelings may be camouflaged, and expressed only indirectly. He may deny having any concerns, or even deny that he is ill. On the other hand, he may show perplexingly intense concern about some relatively normal or insignificant body function or extreme worry about events at home or at school. He may appear surprisingly fearful that family members are in danger, perhaps imagining them in a car accident as they drive to the hospital. In such instances, his anxiety about himself has been displaced; he is shielding himself from awareness of his own fears.

The youngster may also shield himself from his own feelings by projecting them on others. For example, a little girl facing hospitalization during acute episodes of a kidney disease would declare to her mother, "You just want to get me back in the hospital to get rid of me!" It was more bearable for her to imagine that her mother had such hostile wishes than to recognize her own angry feelings.

Youngsters conceal their feelings from themselves because they sometimes need to. It is generally not helpful to interfere directly with a youngster's denial or displacement or projection by confronting him with the truth of his fear or anger. Children, as much as do adults, need to set their own pace in becoming aware of their inner feelings. Parents, however, may feel less puzzled and upset if they recognize that it is common for children to camouflage their feelings in such ways. Furthermore, the camouflage is a sign that the child is worried and in need of effective reassurance that although he is enduring a difficult experience, he will be helped to deal with it — he will not be abandoned to face it alone.

Helpful Measures

Preparation.   Preparation, beginning before admission and continuing until discharge, is as crucial for the school-age child as for the preschooler. The principles of effective preparation are those described in Chapter 4.

With the school-age child, the use of books or pamphlets written for children facing hospitalization can be more effective. Furthermore, such a child is likely to have greater capacity to think about and discuss the experience directly and realistically. He may profit from a pre-admission visit to the hospital and a chance to meet staff members (as long as he is encouraged afterward to ask questions and express his feelings about what he has observed). However, because of the child's intellectual advances and increasing realism, it is easy to overestimate what he understands. When he is worried, a child's understanding can be impaired, and his mind may be swamped with fears arising from his imagination, just as may the mind of the anxious adult. It is very important, therefore, to be alert for indications that significant information has been forgotten or become confused.

Most school-age children can read a clock. Because they can tell time correctly, it is easy to overestimate their sense of time in preparing them for the hospital. An interval of time, such as one hour, is an extremely abstract idea. In a child's actual experience, an hour may be an instant of pleasure or an eternity of worry. It is helpful, therefore, to make time meaningful by referring to familiar events: "I'm going to the hospital lunchroom for a half hour — that's how long it takes you to watch 'The Flintstones' every afternoon at home." "You will have your nebulizer treatment at 7:30 a.m. — that is, after you wake up in the morning but before you eat breakfast."

In preparing your child for his hospital experience, you will be imparting information. Just as important — perhaps more so — you will be communicating your attitudes. If you feel intensely worried about a procedure he faces, or about a new medication to be used, your child will readily sense your apprehension, and his own fears may be intensified. It is therefore essential to work closely with the hospital staff. You will need, first, to discuss thoroughly your own questions, doubts, and fears with the doctors and nurses, and perhaps with the hospital chaplain or social worker as well.* Second, you may need to ask staff members to help prepare your child for special procedures, since they are likely to be better informed and to feel calmer and more confident about the procedure than you.

Identifying the Sources of Help. The hospitalized child has physical, emotional, educational, social, and spiritual needs. The head nurse or social worker in your child's hospital division can help you and your child learn about and make use of the sources of help available. It may be extremely reassuring to your child to know that there is a special teacher to help him with the assignments his classroom teacher may send in. It may be comforting to know that he could talk over with a compassionate chaplain his questions about why God allows people to become sick. It will probably be cheering to know that there is a recreation room where he can be among other youngsters and perhaps learn new games and skills. It may be a significant source of hope to learn that there are laboratories where scientists are studying more effective ways of controlling his illness.

Helping Your Child to Be Helped. In spite of the excellent resources of many hospitals, children may experience isolation and feelings of abandonment. There are several important reasons why this may happen. First, the child's energy may be drained away by his illness or pain. He may be unresponsive to those around him, and seem not to care if they are present or absent. Therefore, his need for reassuring companionship may be underestimated.

Second, he may be intensely irritable, and outwardly reject the loving ministrations offered him. Parents of acutely ill children sometimes feel a wish to be very, very close to their child — a mother may long to caress, to enfold the child, even to take him again within her own body protectively. Members of the professional staff wish to comfort and to heal. The child's resentment about his illness or his shame about being dependent on others may lead him to respond so disagreeably that parents and professionals tend to feel hurt and to withdraw.

Third, if the child is critically ill, the staff may shrink from developing a personal relationship with him. That is, although they may

---

*Parents often try to settle their doubts by collecting opinions from friends, relatives, or parents of other patients. This usually increases their feelings of confusion and uncertainty. It is more useful to explore your fears with someone who is trained to answer your questions and help you resolve your doubts.

be thoroughly conscientious about keeping his body as comfortable as possible and about giving appropriate medicines and treatments, their own feelings of helplessness and sadness about his condition may influence them to avoid him otherwise.

In any of these instances, there is the risk that your child will feel abandoned and that he will be isolated in a sensory desert — a plain, hygienic room with nothing to look at or listen to or even to think about but his own misery. Your simple presence, or that of a trusted friend or relative, will give comfort. If your anxiety makes you restless, you might ask if a rocking chair is available (or bring your own) and supply yourself with knitting, sewing, drawing materials, or Silly Putty to occupy your tense hands. You might arrange for links with home — a tape recording of messages from friends and family, letters, poems, or stories to be read aloud, photographs and drawings to be mounted within view. You might borrow a collection of mobiles that could be hung, in turn, over the child's bed. Friends wishing to send gifts might be encouraged to pool their resources and send one of the projection boxes that cast ever-changing patterns and rhythms of colored light across the ceiling.

Finally, your child will need opportunities to release his feelings to you or a trusted staff member. He will need reassurance that it is all right to be taken care of when illness makes him more helpless than usual; that it is all right to cry now and then; that it is all right to feel mad. He will need reassurance that even when he expresses his sadness and anger he will be helped not to lose control of his behavior (that is, he won't be allowed to destroy property; he will be protected from hurting himself and others).

Finally, he will need repeated reassurance and specific examples of ways in which he will be able to take a more active role in his own care as his energy returns. If he recognizes that he can work with the nurses and doctors, it is as though he becomes one of the healers himself, and thus his own sense of mastery and strength may be enhanced.

Sustaining Hope.   Youngsters who are critically ill in mid-childhood can, with sensitive and compassionate care, continue to feel well supported even if they must finally die. Supportive communication is an essential ingredient of compassionate care. A child who feels surrounded by a conspiracy of secrecy and silence among the adults, who observes that they evade his questions and avoid listening to his fears, may yield to despair because he feels abandoned to face his destiny in isolation. In contrast, a child who has a trusted adult available to listen and respond to his concerns, one who understands his need for realistic reassurance, may find it possible to sustain hope to the end.

This hope becomes possible because the range of the child's hopes gradually contracts. For example, children with advancing malignancies at first hope for cure and are heartened by accounts of medical research and experimental medications. Gradually their hopes may become modified and centered upon the idea of remission — a period free of symptoms when they can return to home and school. During relapse, hope may narrow further and be focused on the thought that there will be another medication to free the child of discomfort. In each stage, the child usually seeks — and has a right to — reassurance that the doctors have a plan for his care.

As the scope of his hope narrows, so also may the time span of his concerns and the range of his interests contract. Next month is less important than tomorrow, this afternoon, the next hour. There may be a merciful blurring of his awareness. At the end, nothing may matter more than the trusted hand he holds.

Coping with Impaired Health in Adolescence

"And how old is your daughter now?" asked a psychiatrist in a chance meeting with an acquaintance he had not seen for some time. "Almost 12," she said, "and trembling on the brink of adolescence." "Who's trembling?" the psychiatrist asked quizzically, "your daughter or you?" "Mostly me, I guess," the mother ruefully replied.

Many parents nowadays expect their offspring's adolescence to be a period of turmoil — for the youngster and for the family. The expectation is apt to be well founded whether the teenager is healthy or ill.

In simpler societies, a youngster passes from childhood to adult status by enduring a relatively brief ordeal or rite of puberty. In the United States, the transition is prolonged, perhaps lasting a decade. During this period, the youngster is confronted by the confusions and contradictions of the biological, social, and legal definitions of adulthood in our society. At 12 years, for example, a youth is obliged to pay full fare on trains and at the movies, but is accorded no rights in return (to the contrary, although he must pay for an adult movie ticket, he is barred from "adult" films). At 16, he is licensed to drive potentially lethal weapons — automobiles and motorcycles — and is enticed to exercise his purchasing power on credit. In both instances, he is protected from full legal accountability for the consequences. At 18, he may marry without parental consent, and kill or be killed in military combat; but he could not, until recently, vote for his government or, in many states, buy a bottle of beer.

In some states, not until 21 is he accorded full adult status under the law. Even then, especially if he is a student, he may still be economically dependent on his parents and not accountable for his debts.

During this prolonged and contradictory transitional period, major tasks of development challenge the young person. At center is the question, "Who am I?" To find answers, the teenager must discover, understand, and come to terms with his rapidly changing biological self. He must come to terms with his rapidly changing emotional and intellectual self. He must loosen his ties of affection to his family, and form outside emotional attachments that will gradually lead toward the commitment of an adult love relationship. He must outgrow his dependence on parental care and authority, and learn to regulate his own impulses and actions. He must choose a value system, a life-style, and an occupation that will accord him a sense of significance in society at large.

These monumental tasks must be accomplished in a time of rapid social change, at a time when youngsters are besieged by terrifying questions about their own destiny — will there be breathable air, will there be enough food for all humanity, enough space to occupy, will, in fact, human society continue to survive?

The Challenges

The Maturing Body

The central experience of adolescence is rapid, dramatic physical change — growth and sexual maturation. There are changes in size, proportion, and contour — curving of the hips in girls, broadening of the shoulders in boys. Secondary sexual characteristics develop — facial, axillary, and pubic hair, enlargement of the breasts and genitals. The cycle of ovulation and menstruation is established in girls, paralleled by the boy's capacity to ejaculate seminal fluid containing sperm.

A realistic acceptance of the biological self is one major foundation of a mature sense of personal identity. Before this can be attained, the adolescent must discover, again and again, who and what he is biologically. His mental images of his physical self must be repeatedly altered as his body changes. Furthermore, he must cope with the joy and regret, the pride and shame, the hope and despair these changes are likely to arouse.

Small wonder, therefore, that adolescence is a period of absorption in the changing self. It is a time of intense preoccupation with physical characteristics. A teenager longs to be as lovely as a model or a movie star, as rugged as a champion boxer, as tall as a pro basketball player. Crooked teeth, a pimple or frizzy hair may be cause for despair, a despair that reveals how uncertain the young person feels about his physical adequacy.

Adolescence is a period of wild fluctuations in self-esteem. The teenager may judge his body to be revolting, or he may preen and strut like a peacock displaying the full glory of its tail feathers. He may pamper or abuse himself with excess or neglect of hygiene, sleep, or food. The youngster's declaration of independence may be expressed in physical terms: "My body belongs to me to care for as I want."

Rapid physical changes are paralleled by intensifying aggressive and sexual urges. The adolescent must master these in a society that provides too few constructive outlets and sets forth confusing, contradictory expectations. For example, already aroused from within by biological stirrings, the teenager is further titillated by erotic scenes and sounds on TV, in the movies, in magazines, from singing groups. During the 1970's, the see-through blouse, the miniskirt, the hip-hugging jeans have moved from the discotheque to the classroom. A car in the high-school parking lot is used urgently as a between-classes love nest.

During the often prolonged period between puberty and marriage, aroused sexually but moving hesitantly toward the emotional commitment of an intimate love relationship, the adolescent is afforded no fully acceptable, guilt-free outlet for his sexuality. Although it would be natural for the youngster's sexual feelings and urge to love to flow first toward those closest to him — family members — such feelings are so taboo that the youngster scarcely admits them into his consciousness (or he quells them by convincing himself how frumpy and unattractive his parents really are). Daydreaming, collecting magazine centerfolds, or even enjoying safe intimacy through prolonged telephone conversations are likely to provoke outraged protests from his parents. Self-stimulation continues to be widely regarded as shameful or harmful.

Our society espouses no broadly accepted morality, no clear sanctions either for or against premarital sexual activity. In some sectors of society, dating is strictly monitored. In other sectors, even within the same community, parents subtly urge their young into activities with the opposite sex long before the youngster feels ready. Many families, schools, and clubs have capitulated to the pressure of their young for self-determination and have abandoned regulations and curfews. The burden of decision and self-control is thus left almost entirely upon the shoulders of the young, as is the burden of consequences — guilt, loss of self-esteem, and the harsh realities of venereal disease and out-of-wedlock pregnancy.

Similarly, the adolescent must monitor his aggressive urges in a society that seems simultaneously to demand and to condemn physical aggression. Some of its folk heroes are those who can play the roughest and dirtiest ballgame. Yet in daily life, automation and mechanization increasingly deprive the youngster of the simplest, most effective outlet for discharging aggressive impulses — bodily movement.

The Impact of Bodily Disorders.   Adolescence is a difficult time indeed to appear conspicuously different. It is difficult because then the physical self is the object of such interest, curiosity, and concern;

because bodily changes may bewilder the youngster; because there is worry about physical adequacy, both present and future; because, as the youngster strives to loosen his family bonds, the support and approval of his peers is critically important.

The adolescent is apt to suffer at times from a sense of physical deviation or inadequacy, whether the defect is real or imagined, and his anguish may be intense. The youngster with an extended or threatening illness must deal with special circumstances. His physical deviation is likely to extend far beyond the usual "defects" of adolescence: acne, crooked teeth, stringy hair, skinniness, pudginess. His illness, or its treatment, may produce a variety of differences in appearance and bodily functions (see Chapter 5). The adolescent may be especially sensitive to cosmetic impairment, such as the "moon-face," puffiness, and loss of hair that are side effects of certain powerful medicines. He may suppose that such characteristics will make him unacceptable, unlovable.

Unfortunately, there is likely to be a period of several years, especially just before puberty (pages 95-96) and into the early teens, when the youngster's age-mates will probably react with embarrassment and teasing or avoidance. The ill youngster's physical deviations tend to arouse or reinforce his contemporaries' anxieties about their own bodily processes and physical adequacy. It is not until the mid-teens that many youngsters feel secure enough with their own maturing bodies to accept — and feel compassion for — those with physical disorders.

Certain extended illnesses are associated with delay in growth or sexual maturation. Delay of puberty may, in particular, make it difficult for the young girl to develop a realistic sense of her own sexuality, since the sensations associated with menstruation seem to help girls locate and form mental images of their unseen, somewhat mysterious, internal reproductive organs. For girls and boys alike, delayed puberty may intensify the feeling of inadequacy as girl-becoming-woman and boy-becoming-man to which a young teenager is prone. Such delay also may cause the youngster to be left behind by those age-mates who show an early interest in the opposite sex. Delayed sexual development or growth may cause the youngster to be perceived by teachers, coaches, librarians, shopkeepers as younger than he actually is. His sense of dignity may be outraged if he is treated in babyish ways.

In other ways, also, physical disorders impose special problems for the teenager. Just at a time when the youngster is likely to be feeling an increased sense of modesty, his bodily privacy may have to be violated repeatedly by parents, nurses, and doctors. They may need to inspect, examine, and manipulate his body, and to show an embarrassing interest in his urine, stool, blood, or sputum.

Just when he is struggling to repudiate his affectionate attachment to his parents (freeing himself to form future love relationships), his disorder may require him to submit to intimate bodily contact, such as massage or rectal irrigation. Such procedures may produce pleasant or exciting sensations that are disturbing to the youngster.

The teenager himself tends to alternate between pampering his body and neglecting or abusing it. Such extremes tend to make the management of a disorder more complex and precarious.

The disorder may result in limited bodily movement, either because there is weakness or fatigue or because exertion results in disagreeable symptoms, such as faintness, shortness of breath, or severe coughing. The disorder may result in reduced opportunities for interaction with other youngsters. In either case, the intense longings and drives of adolescence cannot as readily be discharged either through patterned physical activity (such as a hard tennis game) or through casual encounters and permitted intimacies (for example, dancing) with contemporaries. The youngster may, therefore, be prone to explosive release through "babyish" tears and tantrums that embarrass and shame him.

Alternately, the stored-up energies may be channeled into prolonged and vivid daydreaming and perhaps a more-than-usual interest in pornographic magazines. (All teenagers daydream, and most pass through a period of interest in "sexy" pictures that does not, as many parents fear, mean that the youngster is oversexed.) There is no exact way of measuring the amount of daydreaming that contributes to rich imaginativeness and creativity as compared to the amount that obstructs sound emotional and mental development. However, if daydreaming absorbs so much time and energy that there is little available for social interaction and real accomplishments, this may well be considered a sign of emotional disarray deserving professional attention.

Self-control is a particular concern for a teenager. It can be especially worrying if his illness involves episodes of faintness or dizziness, seizures, or periods of unconsciousness in which self-control is totally lost. The teenager wonders — but is often afraid to ask — how he behaves and appears to others during such episodes. Does he seem grotesque or disgusting? Does he make strange sounds or speak foul language?

Finally, the teenager has a newly developed capacity to imagine the future and to understand the meaning of permanence. Therefore, he may experience considerable concern about how his disorder will affect his manhood.

There is a great deal that can be done to help the teenager come to terms with his bodily affliction. However, to be effective such help must also take into account another major drive of adolescence, the drive toward independence.

Striving for Independence

A major task of adolescence is to loosen the bonds of dependence and affection between the youngster and his family of origin. "Who needs parents?" is his belligerent but wistful cry as he strives to quell his longings for protective care in preparation for establishing an autonomous role in society and for forming a new family unit.

Like the young stag that rubs the velvet off his antlers against the trunk of a tree in a forest — and then tests their strength in jousting — so the maturing young human confronts and challenges the authority of his parents. He asserts his own wishes. He may seek physical distance from the household. He may establish a time rhythm in complete disharmony with the family — staying up while others sleep, staying in bed when others arise. He may manifest his individuality by challenging and opposing family preferences concerning bodily cleanliness, hair style, dress, and eating habits.

Unlike societies in which child care responsibilities are shared by kin and older siblings, by nannies (as in England) and metapelets (as in Israel), in our society the responsibility is assumed almost exclusively by parents (aided, sometimes extensively, by the ubiquitous television set). Therefore, it is the youngster's parents that bear the primary brunt of his rebellion; its impact is not dispersed among his kin or other caretakers.

When he breaks his emotional bonds to his parents, in a sense he loses all. Therefore, his wish for independence may well be paralleled by another wish (usually unacknowledged) to retain his position in the family. His sense of loss may cause him sadness; his contradictory longings may make him irritable and defiant.

To convince himself that his family attachments are undesirable, and to become "his own person," he is likely to criticize, denounce, devalue all that his parents stand for. Their stature and weight, style of makeup, mode of dress, way of speaking, occupation, personal value system, and political beliefs all come under fire. At the same time, the teenager experiences a desperate need for substitute relationships, and readily develops crushes on older persons as well as intense and loyal attachments to a group of age-mates.

Loosening ties to the family is a developmental task with a somewhat uncertain outcome. If the family authority and control the youngster confronts seem unyielding, overwhelming — and he feels no confidence in his own strength — he may give up in hopelessness. Alternately, he may express his angry frustrations in explosive protest or acts of destructive rebellion.

However, if the challenge is removed, if parents capitulate, if the opposition collapses, the teenager is left at the mercy of his own powerful drives while his judgment and capacity for self-regulation are still immature. Without outer boundaries to safeguard him, he must be fully responsible for all he feels and does. He may feel unprotected and anxious.

Therefore, neither parents who are rigidly authoritarian nor those who "cop out" or play the buddy role (mother in a miniskirt, father with hair to the shoulders) serve their teenagers well.

Independence and Bodily Disorders.   Control over his own body and over his physical activities is a major focus of the youngster's struggle for independence. "Don't bug me" is his refrain. A physical disorder, however, may necessitate supervision of his diet, sleep, exertion, even his bathroom habits. A 13-year-old with cystic fibrosis reflected about how a boy like himself feels:

> "He's disgusted . . . because he wants to live a life the way he wants to. You know, he has to take his medicine and all that, but let people leave him alone so he can do what he wants." [Doctor asks: "What kinds of things do people bug him about?"] "Well, don't overexercise yourself and don't run too hard, don't play too hard, come home in five minutes, don't stay out too long, and all that other stuff." [Doctor: "What is it that people worry about that would happen to him?"] "He'd probably keel over and fall down in the road some place."

Being "bugged" frequently may arouse resentment if the youngster feels that his capabilities are not respected, his judgment not trusted. It may also arouse chronic anxiety about his own safety.

Even parents of healthy children experience sadness, a sense of loss, and anxiety (along with pride and satisfaction) as their children grow up. It is difficult and emotionally painful to hand over the reins of control at an appropriate pace. For parents of youngsters with potentially serious disorders, it is agonizingly difficult. Again and again, these parents must ask themselves the question, "Isn't the quality of my child's life as meaningful as its duration?" as they strive to find an effective balance between maintaining supervision and granting independence.

"What's the use?" a youngster may wonder if he imagines (rightly or wrongly) that the likelihood of ever becoming an independent adult is uncertain. "What's the use?" his parents may wonder if they expect his life span to be shortened or believe that he could not survive without their care.

"The use" is that any existence not directed toward a goal is meaningless. "The use" is that a youngster without some feeling of self-determination feels anxious and angry — he lacks self-respect. "The use" is that parents won't be around forever. "The use" is that effective medical care may enable him to achieve a venerable old age.

What Will I Become?

From early childhood — when the child plays out the roles of jet pilot, doctor, Good Humor man — through the mid-childhood daydreams of becoming a famous dancer, a statesman, a champion at sports, children explore the question, "What will I become?" In adolescence, the question becomes more realistic and more urgent since the youngster's goals both shape and are shaped by his educational experience, intellectual attainment, and emotional commitments.

The teenager seeks a sense of significance that gradually extends beyond family and peers into society at large. He increasingly interacts with society through wielding his purchasing power, exercising political activism, holding part-time jobs, doing volunteer work. Such pursuits — and the plaudits they earn — help to fill the emotional empty spaces created by the loosening of family ties. Active commitment to various ideals also opens channels for constructive discharge of the adolescent's aggressive and sexual energies. Further, his activities allow him to try out various roles in society before formulating long-range goals.

In our society, the task of choosing a career is complex and anxiety laden. Our societal expectation of upward mobility often denies a youngster the comfortable option of following family tradition, of being a fifth-generation blacksmith or jeweler or typesetter. Rather, U.S. society values individuality and attainment that surpasses that of previous generations — and perhaps thereby repudiates family tradition. Furthermore, U.S. society offers a bewildering array of occupational choices. Some provide an uncertain future, and this makes selection of a career even more difficult. That is, because of rapid social and technological change, occupations that are highly valued today may fail to provide a livelihood a decade from now.

All these social factors both challenge and burden the teenager, whose rapid growth and development is already arousing feelings of uncertainty. A youngster with a physical disorder may, in addition, need to come to terms with the fact that his illness imposes limits on his choice of careers.

Impaired Health and Occupation Choice. In certain occupations, the physical nature of the work would be inappropriate for people with certain disorders. For example, tasks requiring intense exertion or prolonged endurance might be poor choices for those with shortness of breath, weakness or easy fatigability (although a youngster incapable of prolonged effort might indeed be capable of short bursts of intense energy and vice versa).

In certain occupations the work environment would be undesirable. A person prone to fainting spells or seizures would be at high risk in construction work or around machinery. (On the other hand, an apparently undesirable work environment might actually be beneficial. For example, a teenage boy with cystic fibrosis pointed out to his protesting mother that his job in a car-washing shop exposed him to continuous steam, which helped to clear his clogged airways.)

Physical disorders are likely to necessitate absences from the job, either during periods of acute illness or for medical treatment. Such absences are more readily accepted in some occupations than in others.

Firms with mandatory medical or disability insurance coverage are likely to exclude from employment those persons who appear to be high actuarial risks (unless the company can be induced to waive insurance coverage).

The decision where to work must be influenced by the accessibility of medical care. This may pose extensive limitations for the person with a relatively rare or poorly understood disorder, who may need access to a major medical center.

The decision may also be influenced by climatic conditions. For example, it might be undesirable for a heart patient to work at a high altitude. Working in an industrial, smog-polluted city might be hazardous for a person with asthma.

Such considerations may appear almost insurmountable to the young person. Most worrisome, however, may be his uncertainty about his life span. Is it even worthwhile to try to set long-term goals? It may console his family, and help them encourage him, to realize that such doubts are also widespread among healthy adolescents who fear death in military combat or who have become convinced that our physical environment will soon cease to support human life.

A teenager, healthy or ill, who is unable to feel a sense of significance in his society at present and to anticipate finding a meaningful role in the future experiences alienation. He may "thumb his nose" at society through antagonistic confrontations and destructive actions. He may "cop out" and seek a drug-induced euphoria. He may succumb to feelings of hopelessness and depression.

A sense of goal-directedness is crucial for the youth, as it is for the middle-aged and elderly. It is as essential for the physically ill as for the healthy. Even if the illness is a serious one, commitment to safeguard the quality of life must include helping the youngster formulate goals for his personal future. Indeed, medical advances may extend his life to an unexpected degree, and there should be preparation for this possibility.

Helping the Teenager Cope

As parents of youngsters with extended illness stand "trembling on the brink" of their child's adolescence, there are encouraging thoughts to keep in mind. The very fluidity of the adolescent personality, which creates turmoil on the one hand, may be helpful on the other. The patterns of adaptation that have developed during childhood tend to become less rigid, and the youngster can be helped toward more effective ways of coping with life. Furthermore, his intellectual development makes available to the adolescent new modes of problem solving. For ex· ample, he becomes increasingly capable of logical thought and of thinking through solutions to his problems before he takes action. There are, furthermore, many significant ways that parents can enhance the quality of the youngster's daily life and help him cope effectively with the challenge of his physical disorder.

Preparation

Problems that are anticipated can often be ameliorated through thoughtful planning. If a child's disorder has been a long-standing one, many of the measures that helped him in mid-childhood (Chapter 5) also prepared him for effective functioning during adolescence. However, as the teens approach, it is also of especial importance to find out from the doctor whether puberty is likely to influence the disorder, or whether the disorder may influence puberty.

Your youngster's physical status may be expected either to become less stable at the time of puberty or to improve. If the former is expected, you may feel more confident if you prepare yourself and your youngster for the shifting course. For example, a child with diabetes may need additional insulin during a spurt of rapid growth. Furthermore, his fluctuating hormonal status may make it more complicated to maintain good metabolic balance. Unless such changes are expected, you (and your child) may wonder, "Is he worse? Has his illness become more severe?"

However, the information about possible changes is helpful only if you are assured that it applies currently to your own child. Too many parents of children with cystic fibrosis, and many of the youngsters themselves, have dreaded approaching adolescence because years before they were warned that adolescence might be the end of the road. Feelings of hopelessness and despair influenced some such families to abandon the treatment program. Long-range predictions cannot take into account the possible advances in medical knowledge or individual variations in the severity of an illness. It is well to be wary of statistical generalizations: "Only ____% of children with _____ reach adulthood." Perhaps that prediction was true 10 years ago. Is it true today? Furthermore, which statistic is a brown-eyed boy named Jonathan?

It is, however, especially valuable to find out whether there is likely to be a significant delay in your youngster's growth or sexual maturation.* If so, the doctor will most likely evaluate whether hormone therapy would be appropriate or helpful, perhaps in consultation with an endocrinologist.

It is also valuable to determine whether your youngster's disorder is likely to affect his fertility — his capacity to reproduce,† and whether there is a risk that your youngster's disorder might be transmitted to his offspring. In addition, you would need to know if a daughter would herself be jeopardized by pregnancy.

If delay of growth or sexual development is anticipated, it is helpful to steer your youngster — gently and before the onset of puberty — into associations that are likely to remain accepting and enduring. For example, even though a girl may be left behind by the group of schoolmates who begin to date in the early teens, she may continue to enjoy effective relationships with friends in a choral group or literary magazine. A boy may be abandoned by those who jog off to football practice, but he may excel as a sportswriter for the school newspaper.

Although schools offer many such group associations, it is also worthwhile for parents to consider whether their own groups may be helpful and interesting ones for their youngsters. If parents do not belong

*There is, of course, considerable variation among healthy youngsters in the age at which sexual maturation begins, and considerable variations in normal growth patterns.

†Many people are unclear about the difference between impotence (incapacity to experience sexual arousal and orgasm) and sterility (incapacity to conceive or bear children). It is crucial that you, and later your youngster, clarify which, if either, is likely to result from your youngster's disorder.

to a church, club, or recreation center, it may be timely to join in anticipation of their youngster's needs. Unless a youngster feels kinship to a group espousing a constructive goal and value system, he is likely to ally himself with the alienated, the nihilistic — or else to become a loner.

Coming to Terms with Your Feelings

The feelings aroused at the time of diagnosis of your child's disorder — sorrow, regret and guilt, apprehension and anxiety, resentment and anger — are likely to be re-awakened again and again. The approach of adolescence with its expected turmoil, as well as any likelihood of delay or deviation in growth or sexual development, can contribute new worries. You may feel quite uncomfortable about questions concerning menstruation, sexual responsiveness, or fertility. Many parents of today's children straddle the "old" morality and the "new." Although they feel they should be "enlightened," relaxed, and well informed in discussing sexuality with their youngsters, many still experience a residue of the shame and embarrassment that may have been characteristic of their own parents.

To the family that expects its males to be hirsute, muscular and robust, it may be most disappointing to have a son who is frail, slender, and has a peach-fuzz beard. It may seem unbearable to have a daughter possibly incapable of full biological womanliness. It may seem unimaginable for the family line to terminate because the youngster cannot, or should not, bear offspring.

Such feelings are not easily dispelled. It can be helpful, however, to try to recognize them and to air them with a compassionate listener who will understand, not praise or condemn. It can be helpful to remain aware that such feelings may interfere with effective communciation with the doctor about your youngster's sexuality, and to let the doctor (or the nurse) know this is happening so that he can attempt to help you.

It is most essential to understand your own feelings, because your youngster will sense them, even if you avoid putting them in words. A frail boy well knows it if he is viewed as an inadequate weakling by his robust, athletic father — he knows it from his father's facial expression, his tone of voice, his gestures, and the way his father chooses to spend, or not to spend, time with him.

Far better if the father can recognize his disappointment, can reduce the intensity of his feelings by venting them on a trusted listener, can find alternate ways to satisfy his longing for robust, masculine companionship, and can strive to uncover other characteristics in his son that he can value.

Finally, until you can master your own feelings about your youngster's impairment, you can scarcely communicate with him effectively or give him the understanding and support he needs.

Imparting Information

The adolescent's newly developed intellectual capabilities, especially the capacity for logical thought and abstract reasoning, may either help or hinder him in coping with his disorder. He is now capable of understanding complex bodily structures and processes, as well as the effects of disease. Considerable physiological information is available to him through the mass media and the high-school curriculum.

Approaches to explaining his illness that have been useful with the younger child (pages 111-120) and ways of helping him explain to others (page 97) can be useful with the adolescent also. It is not usually appropriate, of course, to use playthings or puppets as vehicles of communication with the teenager. But since teenagers do vary in their capacity to understand purely theoretical or abstract explanations, drawings or models of the human body and its organs are helpful supplements to verbal explanations. There are materials that the doctor, a voluntary health agency, or a school biology department may be able to supply.

Knowing is a way of feeling in charge. Many an adolescent shields himself from anxiety by taking an intellectual view of his disorder. He may become absorbed in learning about its physiology, treatment, and relevant scientific research. In some cases, however, the youngster's capacity to understand the disorder intellectually is well ahead of his readiness to accept it emotionally. If he seeks, or is exposed to, information he is not ready to assimilate, his anxiety may be heightened. Therefore, it is essential to allow the teenager to set his own pace in seeking information and, usually, to take the initiative in asking questions. However, he does need assurance that it is all right to ask, and that there are people both willing and qualified to answer.

Because of the adolescent's intellectual advances, his family and medical caretakers may readily suppose that his understanding of his disorder can be entirely rational. This is rarely, if ever, the case. Even intelligent teenagers who have been carefuly educated about an extended illness, such as diabetes, tend to construct personal theories about their disorder. These theories blend fact, fancy, and emotion; they reflect the youngster's life experience and image of himself and of his place in the world. Furthermore, most, if not all, teenagers blame themselves (at least in part) for their illness. A common idea is that the body has been damaged by sexual activity, particularly exploring or manipulating the genitals. If the self-blame is intense, the illness may be interpreted as deserved punishment, and the youngster may experience feelings of unworthiness and hopelessness.

However, even though the teenager will absorb and interpret information in a highly individual way, it is nonetheless important for factual information to be given. Information can help to keep distressing fantasies within bounds and the youngster's theories somewhat attuned to reality.

The trust of the adolescent is often more fragile than that of the younger child. He quickly detects phoniness, the meaningless platitude. Therefore, honesty in informing him about his illness is essential. However, honest information should be given in doses he can assimilate. Honesty should never close the door on hope. Every youngster needs reminding that there are things being done on his behalf, by him, his family, his doctors, and by research scientists.

His sexual maturation is an area of crucial importance and special sensitivity for the teenager. Informing him, therefore, that puberty may be delayed (or will not occur without hormone therapy), that he is incapable of reproducing, or that he risks passing a dangerous disorder to his offspring requires tact, compassion, and a delicate sense of timing. If possible, the timing should be determined by the readiness of the youngster to come to terms with the information rather than being determined by the urgency and anxiety of parent, doctor, or nurse ("Let's get it over with"). If puberty is expected to be delayed in onset but normal in character, it may be wise to inform the youngster during the preteen years, when, hopefully, he is being given other information about human sexuality and reproduction. A youngster who is unaware that his contemporaries will probably mature sexually before he does is likely to conclude that he is deficient when they surpass him. Further, he will need support in expecting and dealing with the tendency of outsiders to treat him as though he were younger than his age. It will help him to know that you understand that this hurts and angers him.

There is no ideal time to transmit information as potentially devastating as the likelihood of sterility. Society is slowly recognizing that adults who do not have children can nonetheless lead meaningful lives, and may even, in the view of some, be making a positive contribution by *not* adding to the world's teeming population. However, most young people do wish to have the opportunity to make their own choice about reproduction. Being deprived of this choice can threaten the adolescent's sense of adequacy and of self-determination.

It has been found that if information about probable sterility is given in early adolescence, either it may seem so remote and abstract that it is meaningless for the youngster or it may be emotionally overwhelming. Therefore, it may be wiser to proceed one step at a time and to wait until sexual maturation is established. The older teenager will also have more available pathways toward compensatory gratifications — perhaps preparing for a vocation that involves nurturance and caretaking (as do the health and teaching professions). In any event, it is essential that the youngster understand that the capacity for sexual arousal and gratification is not related to sterility.

If there is a risk of passing the disorder to offspring, it is not enough simply to supply the youngster with information about the percentage of risk. He needs careful guidance in regard to premarital intercourse and the chance of pregnancy. He needs to know that when the time comes to consider reproducing, his decision about it will be a complex one, and it will be governed by attitude and emotion as much as by reason. (Most of the issues explored in Chapter 7 will apply to him also.) He needs to know that there will be counselors available to help him and his future mate reach a thoughtful and personally meaningful decision.

These sensitive issues will be painful and complex for you as well as for your teenager. You may find it helpful, in planning how and when to bring them up for discussion, to consult with a physician specializing in adolescent medicine or a psychiatrist experienced with children and young adolescents.

All such information concerning sexual development and adequacy is difficult to absorb. Many youngsters can assimilate it only little by little. They will have periods of avoiding the facts and denying their reality or of forgetting what has been said. These are common ways of warding off emotional pain, and it is usually wise to respect the youngster's own pace in learning about himself.

Fostering a Sense of Kinship

Fully as much as the younger child* and perhaps more so, the adolescent needs to associate himself with a group of contemporaries. Classmates, teammates, neighborhood or street-corner gang, kids from the church congregation, country club, and recreation center, co-workers after school at the supermarket, hospital volunteers — he may feel a bond with any such peers.

Within his chosen group, he finds support and kinship as he strives

*Chapter 5.

to gain independence from his parents. These friendships fill the emotional empty spaces created as family ties are loosened and provide way stations as the youngster moves hesitantly toward the emotional commitments of adulthood. His experience and personal growth are enriched as he is exposed to new modes of behavior and value systems. Even during periods of acute illness, interactions with his contemporaries help to prevent an exclusive self-absorption and preoccupation with his inner sensations and worrying thoughts.

Most teenagers with a significant bodily disorder experience deep fears of rejection by their contemporaries. This is true whether the illness is a newly acquired one or a long-standing one. There is some realistic foundation for such concern. Alterations in a youngster's physical appearance or obvious symptoms of illness are likely to arouse discomfort in his contemporaries, especially during the early teens, when they, too, are feeling anxiety about the changes within their own bodies. It can be most supportive to a youngster to let him know you realize that his physical problems may make others feel embarrassed sometimes and that their reactions will upset him. It is supportive to explain that their embarrassment is partly a reaction to their own disturbing bodily development, and that by the mid-to-late teens, almost all youngsters become much more understanding and tolerant of differences. They are then likely to sympathize with the failures of an acquaintance with a medical problem, give him credit for his efforts, and praise his successes.

Your teenager may work hard to keep a cheerful grin on his face in the company of his peers. He needs encouragement from you not to keep his emotions bottled up all the time. His feelings of worry, resentment, or shame need to be confided to someone he trusts. If he cannot talk about his feelings to his parents, he needs access to a trusted relative, friend, teacher, counselor, or minister. You may need to make sure he has opportunities to talk with such a person.

You may also wish to find out from your child's doctor or the appropriate voluntary health agency* whether there are group experiences available for youngsters with the same disorder. In some medical centers, professional personnel (doctor, nurse, social worker — or a team of such persons) conduct group discussions for adolescents with health problems. Special camping programs are at times available for youngsters who share certain disorders, such as diabetes, cystic fibrosis, and hemophilia. Special recreational and sports programs are available in some communities, run by a rehabilitation or recreation center. All such programs may offer three significant benefits: exposure to other

*See Appendix.

youngsters who cope with similar problems and may have found effective solutions; an opportunity to share the emotional aspects of such problems (such sharing often lightens the burdens and reduces the sense of being alone in misery); an opportunity to develop new skills.

It is worthwhile considering whether your own home offers a welcoming and attractive gathering place for your youngster's contemporaries. Is there a place for private rap sessions, listening to the radio and records? Is there some simple but appealing sports equipment — a basketball net, a baseball pitchback, tennis backboard, archery set, Ping-Pong table? Is there a fireplace or grill for toasting hot dogs and marshmallows?

During periods when your youngster's illness is more severe and his energy at a low ebb, access to a telephone may be crucial in keeping him in contact with his contemporaries. A phone extension that he can use in private may be, literally, his line to the outside world. However, prolonged use of it may create inconvenience or resentment in other family members. If the teenager agrees that his phone calls will not interfere with responsibilities such as homework, and if the family income can absorb the expense, a separate line for the youngster's use can be of great value.

Your teenager may need help in disclosing information about his disorder effectively. He, as much as the preteen, is likely to feel "good inside" if he can share his "secret" with a trusted buddy (See Chapter 5). However, if he blurts out information in ways that are embarrassing or frightening to his contemporaries, they may respond with teasing or avoidance. He is likely to benefit from an opportunity to rehearse some simple explanations he could make when others wonder about his medication, his treatments, or his symptoms.

Some teenagers are able to use humor or irony effectively. Barry, for example, faced the difficult adjustment of transferring to a new high school when his father changed jobs. Barry was conspicuously small because of his medical disorder, and realized that the kids would surely notice and respond to this. Therefore, on the first day, he went in with a smile on his face (though quaking inside) and declared, "No autographs until after two o'clock today, kids!" The others were able to share the joke with sympathy, and admired Barry's cool.

The parent of the teenager can work in cooperation with significant school personnel to insure that the expectations of the staff are realistic, that your youngster is not needlessly exposed to physical hardship and embarrassment, and that every opportunity for constructive accomplishment is made available. (Many helpful ways of doing this have been described in Chapter 5.)

Furthermore, your youngster's physical differences can be somewhat minimized. For example, the teenage girl whose bodily maturation is delayed need not endure the embarrassment of wearing a childish undershirt long after he. friends are wearing bras. At least one manufacturer has pioneered in styling bras for the flat-chested young girl that can be contoured with padding, and then conform to her shape as she develops.

Shopping for clothes can be distressing, especially if the mirror in the dressing room reflects an image of clothing that looks grotesque in style or size. However, a teenage girl of short stature no longer must wear clothing styled for the child. She now has a choice of more sophisticated but properly proportioned junior petite sizes. (In fact, clothing manufacturers are beginning to take an interest in the special clothing needs of persons with special physical needs — a group that comprises an enlarging proportion of U.S. consumers.)

Many teenagers prefer shopping alone or with a friend. It can be helpful if a parent does some advance scouting to be able to tactfully suggest shops or sections of department stores where the selection is likely to be appropriate. For a son, who is likely to dislike shopping for clothes anyway, the parent can help by bringing home a selection for him to try on in privacy.

Youngsters with skin disorders can choose among a number of preparations effective in healing or masking the flaws. Youngsters of both sexes who experience hair loss (a problem associated with the use of certain powerful medications) have a wide choice of hairpieces and wigs.

Adolescents experience tentative intimacy with each other in many physical ways — in wrestling and suggestive dancing-without-touching, for example. They experience intimacy through food sharing — to the extreme, occasionally, of a group's munching the same apple in turn or of one taking chewed gum from her mouth and popping it into the mouth of a friend. Therefore, if a special diet is needed,. it should be managed so as to permit the youngster to participate in shared food experiences as much as possible.

A teenager whose carbohydrate intake was restricted enjoyed carrying out the role of food provider for the group. On almost any pretext, she baked a cake or batch of cookies for her friends, and thus shared the food experience without actually eating herself. She reduced her own sense of deprivation, however, by baking a flavor which, although well received by others, was not one she especially liked.

Finally, it is helpful to remind your youngster (and yourself) that although he feels different from his contemporaries, they are, in fact, *all* different from each other. Teenagers outwardly symbolize their kinship through hairstyle, mode of dress, private language which assigns new meanings to old words, ritual handclasps, shoulder punches, finger gestures. Inwardly, they often feel alone, strangers to their families and to themselves with their rapidly changing bodies, emotions, ideas, and value systems. Some mature rapidly and some more gradually. Within an individual youngster, intellectual, social, emotional, and bodily maturation may each proceed at a different pace. Some youngsters involve themselves early with the opposite sex, some late. Therefore, within most U.S. communities there is such variability among adolescents that almost any youngster should be able to find others with whom he can develop a sense of kinship.

Developing Effective Teamwork

Developing effective teamwork among parent, child, and doctor requires tact and understanding during the preteen years,* and it is likely to be even more complex during adolescence, in part because parent (and doctor) may be misled, bewildered, and upset by the youngster's contradictory child-adult behavior. Furthermore, just in a period when the youngster needs independence, his disorder may become more difficult to regulate (because of the physiological changes of adolescence).

Physical contact with their parents is embarrassing for many teenagers. They may respond to a treatment involving bodily closeness with giggling, squirming, or frank avoidance. Supervision of diet, medication, and activity may be interpreted as snooping, prying, bugging. It may arouse resentment and defiance.

For these reasons, it is desirable to encourage the teenager to assume increasing responsibility for his treatment. If there are certain maneuvers he cannot carry out alone (postural drainage, for example), he may accept help more comfortably from one parent than from another or from a more distant relative, a friend, or a neighbor. His parents may be able to arrange for such help by offering a compensatory service in return.

Although independence should be encouraged, the youngster may feel deserted and frightened if supervision is stopped completely. For example, a 17-year-old boy with a serious disorder involving excessive copper in his system insisted that his mother put his pills out for him every morning. He seemed to need this simple gesture to reassure him of her concern and willingness to share responsibility.

Teenagers vacillate in their capacity for independence. Parents

*Chapter 5, Managing the Medical Regimen.

often feel "damned if I help, damned if I don't." Because the parent-adolescent relationship is likely to be troubled at times, it is essential that a teenager have direct and private access to a doctor who is capable not only of treating the physical aspects of his illness but also of listening to his fears, worries, and questions. (If the doctor is not comfortable in this role, perhaps he could refer the youngster to an appropriate medical or nursing colleague.) An increasing number of physicians set aside special hours for adolescent patients and encourage them to make and keep their appointments independently. Although valuing such opportunities, the teenager may utilize them erratically. Most adolescents still have need for their parents to stand by supportively. With typical inconsistency, a teenager who spends hours on the phone with his peers may panic at the idea of calling a doctor's office. If he is worried about himself, he may genuinely need a parent to accompany him to the medical center or office.

Furthermore, it is still essential that parents have periodic private conferences with the doctor. The adolescent has the right to some confidentiality, so parents should not expect the doctor necessarily to report the attitudes and emotions the youngster has expressed. It is necessary, however, for parents to keep informed of his physical status and treatment needs. It is helpful to know what explanations the doctor has given the youngster about his condition. It can be useful to let the doctor know what questions, fears, and hopes the youngster expresses at home. Finally, parents need an opportunity to express their own questions, fears, and hopes.

Managing a Diet

Food is likely to have more significance during adolescence than at any other period since the preschool years. The adolescent's contradictory feelings about himself are readily expressed through his eating behavior. He may pamper or abuse his body through his diet. He may thumb his nose at nutritional principles that symbolize adult authority and gorge on potato chips and cola. He may reject favorite family dishes as a way of rejecting parental care. On the other hand, he may eat excessively as though to console himself for the loss of his tender attachment to his parents. He may seek intimacy with peers by sharing food. He may seek new experiences by savoring new gustatory sensations.

Parents, especially the mother, who is usually the provider of food, find themselves aroused by the adolescent's eating behavior. Supervising his food intake is one way of maintaining some control over him and trying to avoid the sorrowful realization of his diminishing need for parental care. The youngster's often blunt refusal ("Yech!") of a dish lovingly prepared may seem like rejection of the parent's affection.

If diet is an important aspect of the medical regimen, as, for example, in diabetes, kidney disease, and obesity, parental supervision is appropriate. However, if parents engage in excessive and seemingly mistrustful checking up, the youngster may respond with defiance. In contrast, parents may feel unbearably guilty about withholding certain foods, and give in to the youngster's beseeching ("Surely a *taste* won't matter!").

Food is so emotion laden for both parent and teenager that dietary regulation can become one of the most troublesome aspects of illness. Trying to understand the attitudes and feelings aroused can be one of the most constructive steps a parent can take. It can be relieving to express some of his own feelings directly to the teenager: "It makes me feel very mean not to let you have french fries — but I care very much about you, and I'm not willing to give you something that would upset your health."

It is essential to clarify with the doctors which foods would actually endanger your child and which would cause only temporary discomfort. In the second case, he may agree that your teenager should be allowed to exercise his own judgment, weighing the risk of a stomachache against the pleasure of sharing a pizza with the gang.

It is essential that your teenager be able to discuss his diet directly with a somewhat detached third party, most likely his doctor, a nurse, or dietitian. It is usually more comfortable for a teenager to accept authority from an adult outside the family. Nonetheless, he needs awareness that his parents are not abdicating — they will stand by to help provide for his needs and to help him endure necessary deprivation.

Dealing with Denial

Hoping that they are invincible, but fearing that they are not, most adolescents test themselves. Some seek constructive challenges; some play with fire in drag races or by drug abuse.

Youngsters with impaired health may play the same game by refusing or forgetting medication, cheating on their diet, purposefully overexerting. Through such behavior, they are saying, "I refuse to acknowledge my illness. I deny my need for medical care."

A host of reasons may underlie such denial — an intense need to assert independence and test adult authority; guilt about burdening the family; feelings of worthlessness; a sense of hopelessness. The behavior is a signal that the feelings, whatever they may be, have become unendurable.

Not surprising, the typical response of parents and doctors is to reason with the youngster, explaining again his need for treatment, urging him to comply, and perhaps reminding him of the seriousness of the disorder. Such an approach frequently backfires. It may intensify the very anxiety and guilt that impelled the youngster to deny his illness.

Overburdened parents sometimes capitulate. Out of their own weariness, resentment, and feelings of futility, they may say, for example, "It's your life, Kenneth," leaving the youngster at the mercy of his inner turmoil (and exposing themselves to intense remorse if the child becomes more ill).

It is far more constructive if you, the parent, can avoid both battling and capitulating. It is constructive to tell the youngster that you are unwilling to accept his denial since you do care about him deeply and then to seek help from a mental health professional. Your youngster urgently needs opportunities to release and understand the feelings underlying his behavior. You may have similar needs.

Desperate Clinging

Some parents of healthy teenagers feel grieved and anxious as their young prepare to leave the nest. Parents of youngsters with impaired health may experience panicky feelings at the thought of the youngster's moving outside the orbit of their protection. Attending school may seem unbearably hazardous even when the doctor feels it is appropriate. Some parents encourage their young to remain at home, believing that this offers protection against such dangers as overexertion and infection.

Teenagers tend to be preoccupied and somewhat worried about their physical well-being. The teenager with a physical disorder may be especially anxious about and absorbed in his bodily sensations, even if his disorder is under good control. Such a teenager may readily capitulate in the face of parental anxiety, become increasingly fearful of physical or social activity, and yield to the parents' wish for him to stay home.

Such a situation is likely to become a tragedy. Each day tends to become a void, without purpose, without commitment to the future, and filled with anxiety and despair. Once such a pattern has developed, it is difficult to change; it is almost certain that urging parent or youngster to behave differently will have little effect. Nonetheless, any relative, friend, or professional person who can win the family's trust should make every possible effort to help them find other ways of expressing their anxiety, and thus perhaps to loosen a little their frantic clinging.

Fostering Independence

Parents often find it hard to recognize the capabilities of their teenagers, especially those with medical disorders.

Although Carol was 14, her parents felt extremely uneasy about leaving her alone in the house during the evening unless her older sister was home. Carol was small, rather frail, and sometimes short of breath, although in no danger of losing consciousness. A favorite pastime when her parents were out was to bake a cake. Her mother feared that Carol might drop the heavy mixing bowl and cut herself, or fall dangerously as she clambered up on a stool to reach the grocery cabinet. Only in talking over her fears with a social worker did the mother realize that, in very simple ways, she could promote Carol's safety while allowing her to be home alone. The heavy mixing bowl could be replaced with a lightweight stainless steel one with a handle; the mixer could be set on the counter, and the ingredients laid out before the parents left the house.

Since the youngster with a physical disorder is sometimes highly dependent on adult authority and care for his bodily well-being, it is especially important to help him find areas in which he can make decisions and function with some autonomy.

In our society, which tends to measure success in terms of money earned, it can be extremely satisfying to a teenager to have an independent income. If his physical condition permits it, he might mow lawns, rake leaves, shovel snow, have a paper route, walk dogs, or baby-sit. (He may, if he looks small or frail, need your help — or a letter from his doctor — in winning the confidence of his first customers or clients. Thereafter, a recommendation from a satisfied client should help him find new ones.)

If paying jobs are difficult to find, he can gain a sense of independent accomplishment by doing volunteer work, perhaps in a library, veterinary hospital, or medical center. Such efforts can yield letters of recommendation that can be valuable later in seeking either a paid job or admission to college.

Adolescents need to attain physical distance from their families from time to time. In the United States, the automobile plays an important role (perhaps excessively so) in symbolizing power and status and in enabling the youngster to achieve physical independence. Earning a driver's license is one of the important rites of passage from childhood to adulthood. Unless there would be physical danger — from seizures or faintness, for example — driving a car can be intensely meaningful to the physically impaired youngster.

Whether or not he drives, his feeling of confidence away from home can be increased if he carries essential information about his disorder on his person. Should he be in an accident, or become ill among strangers, such information could be lifesaving. Identifying bracelets are available for just this purpose from Medic-Alert.

The adolescent has a newfound capacity to think about abstract ideas and values. Therefore, he can also strive to become "his own person" through intellectual and spiritual questioning and discovery. He can exercise self-determination in selecting areas to be explored in high-school courses, workshops or independent study. Unless he shares with his family a secure religious faith, he might be encouraged to attend services in churches of various denominations. He might, through reading and dialogue, explore a variety of beliefs. This may be of immense significance to a youngster who seeks to find meaning in his illness.

Shaping Realistic Goals

The range of life goals possible for young people today is immense. In addition to the effort to insure that persons from all economic and ethnic backgrounds have fair access to educational and vocational opportunities, a wider range of choices has been made available to persons of both sexes. For example, the male nurse and female doctor are increasingly respected for the contributions they can make to society. It is likely that, in time, discrimination against those with physical impairments will become widely outlawed. Federal and some state legislation is reflecting movement in that direction.

The opportunities that society makes available to its young play a part in shaping their destiny. Just as crucial, however, is the young person's belief that he is capable of making a significant contribution to society. Studies of adult hemophiliacs, for example, have shown that the afflicted person's view of himself as employable or not is more crucial than the severity of his illness in determining his adult status in society.

The adolescent's self-esteem has been molded from early childhood by the quality of his relationships to others — first his family, later his contemporaries and significant adults, such as teachers and coaches. Experiences of accomplishment have helped him to recognize and develop confidence in his capabilities (Chapter 5).

With this foundation, early in his teens the youngster begins to need guidance in shaping realistic goals, ones that take into account his capabilities as well as his limitations. He needs guidance in avoiding twin pitfalls: either to deny his limitations altogether and set himself up for bitter disappointment because his aims are unattainable or to overstress his defects and succumb to a sense of futility and hopelessness. He needs the inspiration of learning about others who have had distinguished careers in spite of marked physical impairments. He needs steadfast support in maintaining a sense of commitment to the future.

A successful educational experience is essential, and in many significant ways parents can cooperate with school staff to insure this. The adolescent needs educational continuity. Home assignments are needed when school is missed because of illness. Tutorial help may be needed to enable the youngster to understand concepts explained during his absence.

"Homebound" teachers may be available through the school system, but the adequacy and flexibility of home programs is highly variable. In some communities, a teacher is assigned only after a student has missed an arbitrary number of days or is deemed unable to attend for a predictable future period. A youngster who frequently misses a day or two is unlikely to be eligible for homebound teaching, yet is in danger of becoming gradually overwhelmed as his understanding and accomplishment of his assignments slides farther and farther behind his classmates'.

If homebound teachers are unavailable and the youngster lacks stamina to seek extra help from his regular teachers at the end of the school day, the school staff may be able to recommend qualified teachers in the community who are currently unemployed but interested in using their skills on a voluntary basis. Such teachers — most likely to be temporarily "retired" mothers of young children — might be identified by the school staff or through a community volunteer service bureau. Similarly, a local college or university might (through the student employment office) identify students interested in private tutoring on either a paid or volunteer basis. Even classmates and older brothers and sisters can help.

The youngster can be guided toward realistic goals by vocational counseling. This can profitably be started early in the teens, since the high-school student's choice of courses is partly dictated by his occupational aspirations. In fact, high schools are placing increasing emphasis on career education, including training students in skills that may later become marketable.

An excellent resource is the vocational rehabilitation division of the state department of health (in some states it is a division of the department of education or of labor). Technically, its services — evaluation, counseling, and training — become available only to those 16 years of age and older. In actuality, it may be possible for a high-school guidance counselor to consult with a rehabilitation counselor on behalf of a student with a special health problem. Furthermore, vocational evaluation and counseling services may be available through a private rehabilitation center, such as the many supported by the National Easter Seal Society.

The public — and some medical professionals — tend to think of such services as being appropriate primarily for "crippled" children — youngsters with a visible paralysis or a missing limb, for example. They may be just as valuable for the youngster whose functioning is influenced by such problems as shortness of breath, fainting or dizzy spells, or a tendency to bleed dangerously.

Occupational choices should take into account emotional as well as physical needs. For example, there are many caretaking or nurturing professions that may be profoundly rewarding for the youngster with impaired health. Such professions include teaching, child care, social work, and the health professions, such as medicine, nursing, physiotherapy, occupational therapy, inhalation therapy, nutrition, and dietetics. Such professions, in addition to their intrinsic usefulness, are valuable for the youngster in several respects. First, becoming one of the healers — identifying with them — increases the youngster's own sense of strength. Second, if the youngster's disorder interferes with his or her own capacity to reproduce, nurturance through a profession can provide meaningful compensation. Third, especially in a health profession, the young person tends to work in an environment in which his own affliction is less conspicuous. He may, in fact, serve as an inspiring example to the afflicted patients he helps, and may have a special understanding of their needs.

Every effort should be made to help the young person avoid the discouraging, even defeating, experience of being repeatedly rejected, or even scoffed at, because he may appear frail or too small or too young for the job he seeks. He should be guided in planning the most effective approach, and may wisely provide himself with a letter from his physician that affirms his capabilities. It has been reported that in China today, society finds a meaningful role for every person, irrespective of his limitations or handicaps. Should the United States — the "land of opportunity" — do less?

Through association with a vocational counselor or a rehabilitation center, or both, the young person can be helped to surmount many of the practical obstacles to gainful employment. He may be advised about the most appropriate facilities for the higher education or vocational or professional training he seeks. (Such facilities must not only be geared to his intellectual capabilities, but also provide a physical environment he can function in. A traditional building with heavy doors, long hallways, and staircases can provide insurmountable obstacles to a young person who is weak or severely short of breath.) He may be advised about the firms that are prepared to employ persons with physical disabilities, perhaps waiving mandatory insurance coverage. He can perhaps be supported in persuading a firm to alter its policies. If his limitations are severe, he can be helped to find employment in a protected work environment. Above all, he can be encouraged to think of himself as a significant member of society — as indeed he is.

Hospitalization

Sources of Stress

Hospitalization subjects the patient to stresses that have much in common from babyhood to adulthood. Therefore, the experience of the hospitalized adolescent is not altogether different from that of the child (pages 127-9). The difference lies chiefly in emphasis. In different stages of development, different issues come to the fore and become primary sources of stress.

Loss of Identity. The adolescent's sense of self is in flux, uncertain. Hospitalization poses the worrying risk of loss of his fragile identity. It involves separation from home — his clothes, books, hobbies, mementos, favorite foods, as well as family, friends, and perhaps a pet. Hospitalization involves interruption of his customary routine and activities. His sense of self is anchored in his activities, accomplishments, and relationships at home, at school, among his various peer groups — and thus, in the hospital it may seen imperilled. Furthermore, the hospital is impersonal (his unit number is more crucial than his name), and thus seems to deny his uniqueness.

Loss of Privacy. The hospitalized adolescent is likely to be exposed to embarrassing physical examinations and manipulations. His body may be inspected by persons of the opposite sex, perhaps by an entire group of staff at one time. His excrement may be collected and examined. Sensitive zones, such as the breasts, buttocks, and genitals, may be stimulated by manipulations (rectal temperatures or swabs, enemas, pelvic examinations). Bodily tension and excitement are likely to be aroused, but cannot be easily and acceptably released.

Loss of Self-determination.   The hospitalized adolescent is subject to enforced dependence and passivity. He has little voice in his own destiny; he is dependent on others for expert care. Such a situation is difficult to accept with equanimity. It is in the nature of adolescence to strive for independence. Rather than yield to his occasional longing to be cared for, the adolescent attempts to deny such wishes; and he is likely to experience shame and anxiety about these wishes as well as about the care he actually receives.

The hospitalized adolescent experiences a sense of helplessness and vulnerability. He is vulnerable to the effects of his own illness and feels helpless to control its course. Loss of control over bodily processes is worrying; one of the most upsetting aspects of an enema, for example, is the patient's fear of involuntary expulsion and soiling. Loss of emotional control can be just as disturbing. Many teenagers make an enormous effort to endure physical discomforts with stoicism. As rigid as a West Point cadet at attention, they may not allow themselves even to cry ouch.

Martha, 14, experienced a most difficult day in the hospital. Needing to have several samples of blood drawn from her veins at different hours, and having unusually small veins that were difficult to enter, she had been subjected to many disagreeable needle pricks. Martha seemed quite calm and controlled through her ordeal. She was allowed to return home for the weekend, but expected to reenter the hospital for more tests on Monday. Sunday night, Martha broke down at home and wept uncontrollably. As her mother comforted her, and listened patiently, she learned of Martha's deep fear — not of the discomfort of the needle, but that she might lose control in front of the staff and cry "like a baby." Fortunately, Martha's mother was able gradually to reassure her that the staff would understand, that they knew that even in adolescence (or adulthood) "it's okay to cry when you really need to."

It is because of his fear of loss of control over his emotions and behavior that the adolescent patient dreads anesthesia and powerful pain killers that may alter his consciousness.

The activity of the hospitalized adolescent is likely to be sharply restricted. Whether he is confined to bed, room, or ward, he is unlikely to have available channels for discharge of tension and frustration through activity. To the contrary, his enforced passivity and idleness are likely to increase his self-absorption — his preoccupation with his sensations, his fancies, his fears. Furthermore, he is vulnerable to the misery of other patients, and is likely to fear that his destiny will be similar to theirs.

Fear of Abandonment.   Although the adolescent vigorously resists and denies his dependency needs, he shares with people of all ages a dread of facing alone an unknown destiny. A child who accepts his dependence and an adult secure in his maturity can readily say, "I need you. Don't leave me." The particular poignancy of adolescence is that it is so very hard for the youth to acknowledge his need. He is therefore at rist — at risk that his declarations of independence will be taken altogether seriously, even in the hospital, and that he will be abandoned to endure his fears and his misery alone.

Fear of Deformity.   Bodily strength and beauty seem more highly valued during adolescence than at any other period. Naturally, then, the procedures to which the hospitalized youngster is subjected, as well as the illness necessitating them, arouse fears of distortion, mutilation, or loss of potency. Furthermore, his intellectual development makes it possible for the adolescent to imagine permanence; he thus worries about impairment not only *now*, but *forever*.

Fear of Recovery.   On first thought, it seems absurd to suppose that the adolescent might not rejoice at the prospect of being well enough to go home. His feelings may, however, be more complex. If life at home is turbulent, as is likely during adolescence, he may feel reluctant to leave the relative tranquillity of the hospital. He may feel uneasy about resuming responsibilities, and worry about finding his place again intellectually, socially, and emotionally in his school and among his peers. He may fear that too much (or too little) will be expected of him, or he may fear that he will disappoint himself by being unable to function as he would wish.

Fear of Death.   Although the idea of not-being is an outrage to his sense of self, the adolescent has become both intellectually and emotionally capable of grasping the reality that death involves the total, permanent end of biological life. His own disability, as well as the illness and death of other patients, may arouse this most profound of all fears, whether or not his life is actually in danger.

Responses to Stress

Although the adolescent may respond to the strain and worry of hospitalization in all the ways characteristic of the younger child,* his responses are almost certain to be contradictory and inconsistent because he is in an inconsistent and contradictory period of development. He may shift, sometimes with bewildering speed, between ex-

*Chapter 5.

tremes of rebellious protest (showing restlessness, defiance, rudeness, possibly physical aggression) and yielding compliance (perhaps showing withdrawal into self, loss of interest in surroundings, sadness, feelings of worthlessness and hopelessness).

His understanding of what he observes may be less realistic than usual. For example, a 13-year-old became extremely frightened when he received a blood transfusion. He was able to confide to his mother that another patient had recently died after receiving transfusions. He was convinced she had been all right until the transfusions were started, and imagined that his own transfusion therefore heralded his approaching death. He had overlooked some obvious signs that the girl had suffered from an illness totally different from his own.

His concerns are likely to be disguised, perhaps from himself as much as from others. For example, his anxiety may be displaced from himself to persons and things around him. He may display intense concern and an inappropriate sense of responsibility for a patient he scarcely knows, even while admitting no concern about himself. His unacknowledged longing for home as well as his concealed resentment of professional staff (how could one dare be angry at those who hold his life in their hands?) may be safely released through bitter complaints about, for example, the terrible quality or miserly quantity of the food.

His deepest anxieties are likely to be denied — concealed from his own awareness as much as from others. A critically ill youngster who declares after his return home that the thought of danger "never crossed my mind" is revealing the manner in which he was able to ward off profound fear.

Such denial is sometimes welcomed by the professional staff, who thus feel spared the painful task of listening to the youngster's deepest fears. Opportunity must be available for the young patient to communicate his anxiety when he is ready to, but denial does serve a valuable purpose in protecting the youngster from despair.

It might in fact be said that any mode of response that enables the youngster to endure hospitalization without despair, any mode that enables the professional staff to form an effective relationship with him and to offer concerned and competent care, is a useful way of coping.

Helpful Measures

Adolescent Division.   The adolescent is not a child nor an adult, neither biologically nor psychologically. When he must be hospitalized, therefore, his needs are unlikely to be met with full effectiveness on either an adult division or children's division. Major medical centers are giving recognition to the special needs of the adolescent by developing divisions of adolescent medicine and designating particular units, divisions, or wards as facilities for adolescent in-patient care. Such a division, ideally, is directed by a physician who has specialized understanding of adolescent development. He is likely to supervise patient care in cooperation with colleagues from pediatrics, medicine, surgery, and psychiatry, as well as with the nursing staff. He is likely to cooperate with professional and volunteer workers to insure that the social, spiritual, educational, and recreational needs of the patients are met.

Patients in such a setting are in a milieu in which a sense of kinship with their contemporaries can develop. They are spared the indignity of being among sick children; they are spared the sense of alienation of being among sick adults who may be bothered or annoyed by their behavior and whose own affliction may be frightening to the young patient.

Group Meetings.   The experience of being a patient is more readily endured if it can be shared. The opportunity to voice questions, concerns, fears, or complaints with others in the same boat can be deeply supportive, especially if such group discussions are wisely moderated by a trained discussion leader. It may be most effective if the moderator is a mental health professional — psychiatrist, social worker, or psychologist— who is not directly responsible for the patients' medical care. Sharing thoughts and feelings reduces the sense of being alone; being listened to promotes a feeling of being valued, cared about.

In an adolescent division such meetings may also serve the function of a grievance committee. In fact, if the requests of the patients are reasonable, some influence may be exerted on hospital policy with respect to such matters as bedtime, snacks, telephoning, wearing street clothes in the daytime, and recreational programs. The opportunity to be heard and to take an active role in policy making can significantly offset the feelings of helplessness experienced by adolescent patients.

Although such meetings may develop most naturally in an adolescent division, it may be quite possible with staff leadership to establish a comparable program for adolescent patients who are scattered in various divisions of the hospital. Because of their isolation from their peers, such patients may find a group experience especially meaningful.

In specialized hospitals, in which patients are all afflicted with the same or related disorders (such as a hospital for cancer patients), group meetings that are primarily educational may also be of value. Under a leadership that necessarily includes their physician, young patients can be offered an opportunity to learn more about their disorder, its treatment, and research programs. Those adolescents who choose to attend (some will choose not to) may be able to use such information to contain their anxiety within bearable limits. Generally, they want to know that there is a plan for their care and that there is hope for new treatments. It has been found that they are unlikely to ask for information that would destroy hope.

Effective Relationships with the Staff. Ill adolescents can realistically recognize the hospital staff as people with special competence to help them, a competence not even the most devoted parent could have. The doctor not only makes the diagnosis and prescribes treatment, but he is also the youngster's primary source of realistic information.

As the youngster shares in the knowledge of the doctor (or of other members of the medical staff), he may gain a sense of sharing in the doctor's awesome life-death power. He may imagine himself one of the healers and thus gain a sense of strength within himself.

Doctor and nurse — cooperating with parents — can offer significant support by carrying out a continuous process of preparation. Beginning before admission and continuing until discharge, the patient needs to be apprised, step by step, of what he is going to experience, given an opportunity to express his feelings about it (most likely, ones of apprehension and protest) and invited to ask questions. Such a process reduces feelings of helplessness, and fosters a sense of trust.

A doctor or nurse may become a trusted confidant to whom the youngster discloses worries and fears too painful to reveal to his parents. In fact, the adolescent urgently needs access to a trusted professional who can let him know it is all right to ask any question, but who will leave the initiative to the youngster and allow him to absorb answers at his own pace.

A nonmedical confidant, perhaps the social worker or chaplain, may provide a supportive and private outlet for the release of pent-up feelings about the stressful medical procedures and the staff members who carry them out (since a patient can scarcely dare directly to express anger at the people he so desperately needs). The chaplain may also help the youngster find meaning in his illness, resolving, if possible, the agonizing question, "Oh, Lord, why me?" and striving to relieve any sense of guilt.

It can be distressing for parents to observe their teenagers find strength and solace from persons other than themselves. However, there are few more important ways a parent can help the hospitalized youngster than to encourage him to make effective use of those staff members who are available to meet his needs. Should the youngster face death, the parents, doctor, nurse, social worker, and chaplain will all need each other to share and endure their anguish — and, if the youngster admits awareness of his danger into his consciousness, to let him know that he will be cared for, his pain will be relieved, and there will be a trusted hand to hold when he needs it.

Activity Programs. The intense involvement in *now* that is characteristic of adolescence helps to keep the idea of personal death at a distance. It is important to reduce the adolescent patient's preoccupation with his illness by involving him in recreational activities. Activities that permit self-expression — music, art work, or writing for a hospital newsletter — may offer channels for release of pent-up feelings and for development of new skills and unrecognized talents. Should the hospital be located near a college, students interested in developing recreational programs on a volunteer basis (their age disposes them to an easy rapport with teenage patients) may be readily available.

School assignments, with tutorial help if needed, help not only to keep the patient abreast of his classmates but also to keep alive a sense of purpose and the crucial goal-directedness that gives meaning to life. It is likely that parents will need to work closely with the patient's teachers to design a realistic program.

Bonds to Home. Visits from friends and classmates afford an opportunity to keep abreast of news and keep meaningful relationships alive. Friends can listen to gripes with sympathy and be less upset by them than parents.

It is important for family members to visit regularly. However, such visits may at times be painful for parent and patient alike. It is hard on parents to become the targets of their youngster's stored-up frustration and despair; it arouses guilt and grief when their youngsters cry out, or even just hint, "Why aren't you powerful enough to make me well and get me out of here?"

On the other hand, parents are sometimes so overcome by their sadness and anxiety during visits that there is a reversal of roles. The youngster, the one who should be comforted, finds it necessary to become the one who comforts.

If the emotions on both sides are intense, it may be helpful to introduce a simple activity into the visit, perhaps cards, a board game, or a crossword puzzle. The parent might read aloud a magazine story or newspaper article. If the young patient is very sick and unresponsive, the parent's mere presence is comforting. It is difficult for an anxious parent just to sit. A mother may reduce her tension by knitting or sewing; many fathers, alas, find such outlets less acceptable and find little to help them endure.

Between visits, bonds between patient and home can be maintained through photographs (Polaroid cameras provide a special sense of *now*), written or tape-recorded messages, drawings, cookies (or any medically acceptable food), and through the telephone.

Extending Life

There are some prolonged illnesses in which the youngster comes again and again to the brink of death and through heroic medical intervention is saved. Each time his condition worsens, his family mourns. They feel intense sorrow and regret. They may have sad and frightening dreams of funerals and awaken weeping. They may wonder and worry, "What will the end be like? Will there be pain? Which part of his body will fail first? Will he look different? Will he know?" Their anguish is intense, and they are likely to feel as did one mother who cried out, "How I wish someone could give me an injection so that for a few hours I wouldn't have to think or feel!"

If the youngster's life is saved, his parents may, to their consternation and distress, feel not only relief and joy but also resentment and anger. This ambivalent reaction, which is troubling and puzzling to them and to the staff, is a symptom of emotional overburdening. Having experienced the intense grief of their expected loss, the parents find it almost unbearable to reverse their mourning. Understandably, they may long for an end to their anguish.

The adolescent may experience such longings also. In fact, the question has begun to be asked whether adolescents have a right to refuse heroic, life-extending procedures (such as an organ transplant) that may impose severe suffering and have limited chance for success. The question is complex — agonizing. It deeply disturbs doctors and nurses who are committed to saving life above all else.

Those who value the quality of life as profoundly as they do its duration must consider the question legitimate. It can only be answered case by case, and after the legal, moral, spiritual, and psychological issues have been carefully explored. A central consideration is the capacity of the patient to comprehend the totality and finality of death and to weigh the alternatives realistically. Wise and compassionate counseling is needed to help him in this awesome task, and every available source of support should be sought for him and his family so that they may be at peace with the outcome.

The "Battered" Parent

The Onslaught

To survive — let alone enjoy — the adolescence of their young requires that parents be resilient and steadfast. Unfortunately, the period of the youngster's turbulence often coincides with a period of vulnerability in the parent's own life cycle.

The youngster's physical maturation takes place at a time when many parents are becoming aware of their own declining vigor and fearing loss of their sexual attractiveness and prowess. The youngster's development is likely to arouse admiration and a certain wistful envy. It is likely to revive memories in the parents; long-forgotten desires and fears may again be stirred. Parents locked in a troubled marriage, as well as parents who have been widowed, separated, or divorced, are likely to become poignantly aware of their own unhappiness.

Furthermore, the youngster's challenge of their parental value systems is likely to occur at a time when the parent's own sense of significance is uncertain. Parents may be deluged by a tidal wave of the adolescent's scorn and hostility. Their accomplishments, their style of recreation, their attitudes, political and religious beliefs, personal habits, mode of dress, hairstyle are criticized and denounced — just when the parents themselves are wondering whether their own accomplishments have been worthwhile, whether their life-style is meaningful. Small wonder that they should feel anxious and sad — and angry at the youngster who further stirs up their self-doubts.

The youngster repudiates his need for his parents and strives for independence. The closer the ties have been, the more fervently, in fact, he may denounce them — to his parents' utter bewilderment. He thus faces them not only with the pain of loss but also with the frustration of their natural wish to find some fulfillment through their offspring.

In the United States, where the nuclear (parent-child) family is likely to be separated from kin, parent-child relationships may be especially intense, undiluted by attachments to aunts and uncles, nephews and nieces. Therefore, the turbulence in the family with an adolescent can reach hurricane proportions.

The Influence of Impaired Health

Parents of the healthy adolescent feel resentment and anger (as well as affection and devotion) toward their disruptive youngster.

Parents of an adolescent with impaired health have experienced the emotional, social, and financial burdens of the disorder and thus have additional reasons for feeling some resentment. Furthermore, because they have given so much of themselves in response to the youngster's needs, the adolescent's scorn and repudiation can arouse especially bitter feelings.

However, it is scarcely acceptable to feel resentful, angry, or bitter toward a youngster who is ill. Parents are therefore further burdened by the remorse and guilt their resentment is likely to arouse within them.

Furthermore, parents of an ill youngster are likely to feel intense worry about granting him the independence he may seek. Although most parents spend wakeful hours at night waiting for the return of a youngster who has started driving the family car; although most parents anxiously wonder if their teenager will abuse his body with drugs, alcohol, cigarettes, and the like, parents of an ill teenager can scarcely avoid feeling a heightened sense of risk when the youngster is out of their protective surveillance. And for the single parent, or the parent whose spouse is unwilling to share the responsibility, this sense of risk can seem overwhelming.

Sources of Consolation

It is comforting to keep in mind that early adolescence, the period just before puberty and during it, is likely to be the stormiest, since the youngster is experiencing immense physical and emotional turmoil. By mid-adolescence, when sexual maturity is established, the scene often improves. There is increased hormonal stability (for example, the girl has a predictable menstrual cycle). The youngster is likely to have come to terms with his new physical self. His aggressive and sexual energies are increasingly directed toward activities and persons outside the family. His intellectual maturation enables him to use logic and to deal with some conflicts through dialogue and thought rather than through impulsive action or emotional outburst. Having earlier denounced and repudiated his parents, he may gradually begin to emulate them.

Parents may feel encouraged if they remind themselves that the storms of adolescence will subside. More than this knowledge is needed, however, to maintain an equilibrium in dealing with the youngster. Parents need frequent opportunities to vent the emotional turmoil which their adolescent arouses. If their strong feelings are stored up inside, without an appropriate outlet, they are almost certain to erupt explosively in response to the many provocations an adolescent offers.

Parents need to feel understood and supported by husband or wife, close friends, or other relatives. There must be some warm presence in which the parent can seek comfort and healing when his self-esteem is shattered by confrontations with his adolescent.

If a parent, especially the housebound mother of an ill teenager, has no meaningful existence apart from the care of her youngster, his rejection and criticism and scorn will be unbearably painful. Therefore, it is essential that parents find sources of self-fulfillment and joy outside of the care of their young.

7

Should You Have Another Baby?

Many parents faced with extended illness or disability in their child feel an urgent desire to have another baby. Some seek a way to shield themselves against the pain of possible loss by providing for replacement. Some hope that another child could fulfill dreams that, in the case of the ill child, have had to be given up. Some seek to insure their own continuity through generations to come (and who doesn't have some unspoken longing to leave an imprint on the world through his work, his creativity, or through his children?).

However, the wish for another baby is opposed by the fear of having another afflicted child. A painful state of conflict may be reinforced by friends and relatives, doctors and nurses who have expressed their own opinions from a wish either to offer solace ("You can have another child") or to advise caution ("This is inherited; you should not have any more children").

Your decision about whether or not to have another child is an extremely complex and intensely personal one. Although you may benefit from professional help in considering the alternatives, only you and your spouse can decide the wisest and best course for you. There are, however, several ways to insure that your decision is as sound as possible. First, ample time should be allowed to arrive at your decision. Although a feeling of urgency is an understandable response to the shock of learning about your child's disorder, grief tends to impair judgment. The period of intense grief about your ill or disabled child is probably the worst possible time to make any decision with far-reaching consequences.

Second, it is important to try to understand your own needs and wishes concerning another child. Why is it important to you to have this child; how might it be healing? Would your relationship with this child be jeopardized? Third, you will, unhappily, need to consider whether another child is likely to be afflicted with the same disorder. Fourth, you may need to consider what choices are available to you, such as preventing pregnancy, terminating pregnancy, and finding alternate forms of parenthood.

Risks to the Parent-Child Relationship

For most people, having a child with a serious disorder produces some feelings of inadequacy, even if mild and temporary: one values oneself as a parent a little less highly. Having another child — a healthy child — can be healing, particularly because it may help to restore one's self-esteem.

However, would it be realistically possible to care for another baby as you would wish? That is, are the needs of your ill child likely to absorb most of your time? Would his care drain your energy, so that little would be available for another baby? Could you meet the physical and emotional needs of another child in a way that would be satisfying for him and for you? Would time, energy, and interest still be available for your own personal concerns, and for your marriage?

Could you truly value another baby's uniqueness, his individuality? Or would that baby be expected to fulfill the hopes that had to be abandoned with the ill child?

Kevin had hemophilia. His father was section manager in a large department store. Although he was competent, he was one of many administrative personnel. He enjoyed no particular distinction — in no way did he seem special or particularly admired. His muscular, robust physique was not challenged in any way.

There had been years of special recognition. First in high school, later in college on an athletic scholarship, he was a football hero. Week after week, he enjoyed roars of approval from the crowd in the stadium and the back-thumping, shoulder-hugging admiration of his teammates. Even in his memory the sound of cheers had almost faded now, but it was his secret dream to live out a replay through his son. A hemophiliac play football? No way. How natural, then, that the father should wish for another chance. But what if another son — even if healthy — was not robust and well coordinated? What if he was smart in his schoolwork but a slow and clumsy runner? Would his father not be severely disappointed because the child didn't fulfill his hopes? Would the child be vulnerable to a growing sense of worthlessness because, no matter how he might try, he could never be that which his father longed for?

On the other hand, if another baby was conceived to shield you against loss — and who might not wish for such insurance? — how apprehensive would you feel about him? Would he become unbearably precious, so that it scarcely seemed safe to let him out of sight? Could you allow him to climb a tree, to ride a bike?

To some extent, all parents seek to fulfill their own inner needs through their children, and these questions are difficult to answer. But if you and your spouse are able to reflect about them together, there may be less risk that your relationship with another baby would be excessively influenced by your feelings about your ill child.

Risk of Recurrence

Only a physician can give you sound information about whether there is any significant risk that another baby might have the same disorder as your afflicted child. Such a risk could exist, for example, if you have a medical condition that is known to affect the development of an unborn child. Such a risk is also likely to be present in the case of inherited illness. If inherited illness is present in the family, it is of extreme importance to be sure that you clearly understand the pattern of inheritance (explained in Chapter 8), as well as the chance that each new baby might be affected.

Is it right or wrong knowingly to risk bearing a child afflicted with a serious inherited disorder? There is much controversy over this question. It is quite likely that strong views will be expressed to you by friends, relatives, doctors, and nurses. Some would agree with the views of a thoughtful psychiatrist: "There are things in life to be valued more than bodily or mental perfection; a psychiatrist might choose personality for one. . . . A good society must be able to absorb a few extra defects as the price of freedom."* Others, perhaps particularly impressed with the burden of grief and misery that some inherited disorders may impose upon an affected family, believe that society should attempt to discourage such risk taking. Reaching a decision may be agonizing for you. However, the more freely you can explore your own inner feelings and thoughts about it and the more fully you can inform yourself about available alternatives, the more likely it is that your decision will be a wise one for *you*.

Preventing Pregnancy

Contraception

The most usual alternative to risking a pregnancy is, of course, choosing one of a number of available methods to avoid pregnancy. Information about methods such as rhythm, the IUD (intrauterine device), the pill, the condom, the diaphragm, foams, and jellies may be available

*E. J. Lieberman, "Psychosocial Aspects of Selective Abortion," in *Birth Defects: Original Article Series* 7 (1971): 21.

from your family doctor, gynecologist, or Planned Parenthood Clinic.*

However, information about methods available is not enough. Your own personal characteristics and attitudes are equally important and should be discussed with your spouse and your medical adviser. First, are you basically comfortable with the idea of preventing pregnancy? If the use of contraceptives is in conflict with the teachings of your church or the dictates of your conscience, you are likely to experience uncomfortable feelings of guilt; and you may even try to pacify your conscience by forgetting to use the contraceptive at the crucial time. Second, which method best suits your physical makeup? For instance, in some physical conditions it is unwise to use the pill; some women experience disagreeable reactions to the IUD. Third, which method best suits your personality and your feelings about your own body? For example, perhaps a forgetful person should not use the pill; perhaps a woman who feels uncomfortable about touching her genitals should not attempt to use a diaphragm. Fourth, which method will best preserve a good sexual relationship between man and wife? For example, some men feel that the use of the condom interrupts love making in a distasteful way and reduces sexual pleasure to a disappointing degree; some women feel that the insertion of a diaphragm interferes with a joyful sense of spontaneity in love making; some couples find that jellies or foams make it difficult to stay in intimate contact.

Sterilization

The most certain form of preventing pregnancy is, of course, sterilization. Couples who have completed their families may consider this alternative preferable to using contraceptives for many remaining years of fertility. In the male, sterilization involves blocking (by removal of a tiny segment) of the vas deferens, which is the duct through which sperm pass from the testes to the penis. This is a safe and relatively simple operation that can be performed in the office of a qualified physician. It does not, as many men fear, change a man's sexual capacities, nor his production of male hormone, nor his capacity to have erections and ejaculations.

In the female, sterilization involves tying or cutting the fallopian tubes so that the ovum cannot pass from the ovary to the uterus. Although under certain conditions the tubes may be reached surgically

*If you have difficulty locating a source of information about birth control, you may wish to write the information and education office of Planned Parenthood—World Population (see Appendix).

through the woman's vagina, the operation is usually performed through the wall of her abdomen. This procedure generally requires hospitalization. It does not change a woman's sexual capacities. It does not interfere with menstruation, result in weight gain, nor produce other symptoms of menopause. It does not create frigidity; in fact, many women — freed of the fear of unwanted pregnancy — experience an increase of sexual desire and pleasure.

Currently, sterilization is legal in all states (although Utah permits it only for reasons of medical necessity). In most states it is covered by medical and hospital insurance plans. Although hospital policies do not regulate sterilization performed in a doctor's office, they do govern sterilization of hospitalized patients. Certain church-affiliated hospitals prohibit sterilization for any reason. The majority of hospitals permit it for medical necessity. (Only a minority at present permit sterilization for the emotional, social, or financial welfare of the patient and her family.) Such hospitals usually accept the written consent of the patient and her husband, along with written approval from two physicians (usually gynecologists). A couple considering sterilization can obtain helpful and up-to-date information — as well as referral to a qualified physician if needed — from the Association for Voluntary Sterilization (see Appendix).

At the present time, sterilization must be considered permanent. Two approaches to the reversal, or undoing, of sterilization are being made. First, surgeons are attempting to develop methods of restoring the ducts (fallopian tubes and vas deferens) so that the sex cells can again pass through. However, these methods are not yet entirely reliable. Second, private semen banks are being established. On payment of a fee, a male planning to be sterilized may deposit a quantity of his semen (the fluid that contains the sperm) in such a bank. The semen is mixed with a protective fluid, frozen at an extremely low temperature (this is not a project for the home freezer) and stored. It is believed that this semen can later be thawed and used to initiate a pregnancy. At present, unfortunately, there are many unanswered questions about this procedure. The American Public Health Association Council on Population cautions that it is not certain that sperm frozen for a long period of time retain the capacity to cause pregnancy nor whether sperm that have been frozen are more likely than fresh sperm to cause birth defects.

For most couples, the decision to have one partner undergo sterilization is serious and complex. The man may worry that he would not feel like a truly virile male were he unable to father a child. The woman may believe that she would be less than truly feminine were she unable to bear a child. Either partner may wonder, "What if circumstances should change so that I would later wish to have another baby? What if — through some twist of fate — I should have another spouse? What if a safe and foolproof method is found to predict whether unborn babies are normal? What if a cure is found for this disorder running through our family?" Unless the couple feel certain that they have already had their desired number of children, or unless they both feel convinced that they can find deeply meaningful roles in life through channels other than parenthood, their decision will be difficult. The future well-being of their marriage requires that the decision be one in which the needs, fears, and wishes of each partner are given full consideration.

Interrupting Pregnancy

In spite of the use of contraceptive techniques, unplanned pregnancies do occur. The question of interrupting pregnancy by medical abortion has been subject to some of the stormiest debates in history, concerning as it does man's deepest beliefs about life, about the preservation of the species, about personal freedoms, and about the regulatory responsibilities of society.

The laws of various nations (and of the states in this nation) have reflected a wide range of attitudes about abortion. At one extreme, there has been the position that all abortion — even to save the life of the pregnant woman — is illegal. At the other extreme has been the position that abortion should be available on request. In between these two positions, there has been a wide range of legal grounds for abortion: to safeguard the physical or mental health of the mother; to prevent the birth of babies likely to have been damaged in the womb by maternal illness (German measles, for example) or by medication (thalidomide, for example); to prevent the birth of babies resulting from incest and rape; to prevent the birth of babies unlikely to receive adequate care because of severe disturbance or hardship in the family.

There has also been variation in laws governing the timing of abortion, that is, the period during pregnancy when abortion may legally be performed. (Usually, unless the mother's life is at stake, abortion may be performed only as long as the fetus is considered nonviable, unable to sustain its life outside of the womb.) There has been variation in laws concerning procedures for obtaining an abortion, namely, the channels through which permission must be requested and received. There have been variable laws regulating where an abortion can be performed (such as hospital, clinic, or doctor's office) and by whom (such as physician or nurse-midwife). Finally, individual hospitals have had policies and restrictions that may extend beyond those required by law.

In January, 1973, many state laws restricting or prohibiting abortion became unconstitutional as a result of a significant decision made by the United States Supreme Court. This decision declared, in effect, that any woman has the right, during the first three months of her pregnancy, to decide whether to continue or to terminate the pregnancy. It also declared that, should the woman decide to terminate the pregnancy, the operation must be performed by a licensed physician. Thus, the question of abortion during the first trimester of pregnancy was declared a private matter between a woman and her physician.

The Supreme Court ruled that states are empowered to regulate the practice of abortion between the third and seventh month of pregnancy. Furthermore, state law may forbid abortion after the twenty-sixth or twenty-seventh week of pregnancy, except when abortion is necessary to preserve the mother's life or health.

Opposition to the Supreme Court decision has been manifested in two major ways. First, active attempts are being made to overturn the Supreme Court decision by an amendment to the Constitution. Second, both at the federal and state levels, various efforts are being made to block implementation of the Supreme Court decision by restricting the access of women to financial aid, legal advice, or abortion facilities.

Therefore, a woman or a couple considering abortion must gather much current information: the laws regulating abortion in their own state and other accessible states; the best timing of abortion; the preferred method for carrying it out; whether or not it would require admission to a hospital; length of recovery period; cost (of the procedure, of hospitalization if needed, and of travel to another state if necessary). A family doctor, gynecologist, and Planned Parenthood clinics are valuable sources of information. Should one have difficulty obtaining such information, she may write an inquiry to the national office of Planned Parenthood—World Population.

Understanding a law or a medical program is quite different from considering a reality within one's own womb. Therefore, just as important as the medical and financial information described above is information of a more personal nature; what is the attitude of your church and your family about abortion? Do you accept these attitudes? What are your own intimate thoughts and feelings about interrupting the pregnancy? Have you and your mate shared and come to understand each other's thoughts and feelings about it?

Predicting the Outcome

The question of ending pregnancy by abortion would be less conflict laden for many couples if it were possible to predict whether or not an unborn baby would be normal. New techniques are being developed that promise to do this in certain instances.

Ultrasound is one such technique. High-frequency sound waves (akin to the sonar used in navigation) are directed into the pregnant woman's uterus. As the uterus is scanned with the ultrasound beam, a recording is made of the echoes that result. It is sometimes thus possible to obtain an outline of a particular portion of the fetus, such as the skull. If a series of such scans are made over a period of time, important information might be obtained about the development of the fetal head; for example, a severe abnormality of head size might be revealed.

Amniocentesis is another technique being developed to aid in the identification of unborn babies with severe medical impairments. Throughout its months of rapid and complex development in the uterus, the unborn baby floats in a "bag of waters" that shields and protects it. The bag is termed the *amnion*; the waters are known as the *amniotic fluid*. In amniocentesis, a hollow needle is passed into the uterus, and a small amount of amniotic fluid is withdrawn.

Study of cells found in this sample of fluid may be helpful in predicting whether the baby will be likely to have certain disorders. For example, in Down's syndrome (formerly known as "mongolism"), since the cells are known to include an extra chromosome, chromosome study could reveal whether the unborn baby is affected or not.

Since only a limited amount is yet known about the cell abnormalities involved in many inherited disorders, amniocentesis can give only limited information about certain ones. For example, the pregnant mother of a boy with hemophilia anxiously wonders if the unborn baby is another boy and thus has a 50% chance of having hemophilia also. Study of the sex chromosomes* in the amniotic cells can reveal whether this baby is a boy. Unfortunately, it is not yet possible to determine if the unborn boy is normal or has hemophilia.

In the case of an autosomal recessive disorder, such as cystic fibrosis, it may be possible to determine whether an unborn baby is nor-

---

*Further discussion of genes and chromosomes is found in Chapter 8, under Inherited Illness.

mal. It is not yet possible to distinguish, however, between a fetus that has the disorder and one that has the trait.

The amniotic fluid or cells may also be subjected to a biochemical analysis, such as alphafetoprotein determination. Some alphafetoprotein is normally present in the tissue of the fetus and in the amniotic fluid. However, an abnormally high concentration of the protein offers evidence that there is a serious disorder in the fetus, such as spina bifida, a major abnormality of the central nervous system.

In another special procedure, fetoscopy, the hollow needle inserted into the amniotic sac includes an optical system. This tiny scope may enable the physican to inspect a small part of the fetus through the needle. With skill and good fortune, he may be able to determine if a special area of the fetus is intact or if a suspected defect in its structure is present. He may also be able to obtain a minute sample of tissue from the scalp or a small blood sample from the placenta. These cells can then be examined to determine if the unborn baby is affected with certain blood disorders, such as Cooley's anemia or sickle cell anemia. (This procedure, as well as the other ones described, require a highly trained and scrupulously careful physician, as well as specialized laboratory facilities.)

Rapid progress is being made in this field of prenatal diagnosis, and what is true at the time the author writes this may no longer be true as you read it. Therefore, in considering whether to have another baby, it could be extremely useful for you to inquire if it has become possible to predict through a procedure such as amniocentesis whether your unborn baby would have the disorder that concerns you.

If amniocentesis (or fetoscopy) could be useful for you, when should it be done? As the procedure was being developed, it was learned that early in pregnancy there could be difficulty in obtaining an adequate amount of fluid and living cells. There was also concern that the procedure might cause harm to mother or baby (infection or miscarriage, for example). Results were more successful if the procedure was postponed until early in the second trimester of pregnancy — around the fifteenth or sixteenth week. Fifteen weeks is a long time for an anxious couple to wait, and in actuality the wait may be even longer. Occasionally, the fluid specimen does not contain sufficient cells, and it is necessary to repeat the procedure. Furthermore, to obtain the most information about the cells, it is usually necessary to grow them in tissue culture so that the cells will multiply freely. Laboratory studies may thus take several weeks, bringing one perhaps to the eighteenth to twentieth week of pregnancy.

What Then?

It is unlikely that you, your spouse, and your medical advisers would have planned for amniocentesis if you did not feel willing to act on the results, that is, to permit a medical abortion to be performed should the baby be found to have a serious abnormality. However, the time available to act on the results may be somewhat limited, since it is usually recommended that abortion be performed by the twentieth week of pregnancy. Even more crucial, however, will be your innermost thoughts and feelings about it. Perhaps you reconciled yourself to the idea of abortion early in the pregnancy. Would you feel the same approaching the middle of pregnancy, the time of "quickening" — that first perception of the baby's movement and often the first awareness of the baby's reality as a living being — that is so deeply meaningful for so many women?

If you had already experienced anguish from having a child with a serious disorder, the prospect of repeating the experience could seem unendurable. In such a case, the opportunity to terminate the pregnancy could offer great relief. Alternately, you might decide to carry the pregnancy to term, even knowing that the fetus was probably, or certainly, affected. In a free society, such a choice is rightfully yours, and you would at least have gained a period of time in which to prepare yourself and your family and to plan for the care of the afflicted baby.

Whichever choice is made, it is likely to be a profoundly difficult one for you and your spouse. Some relatives and friends will approve and encourage you, some will disapprove and criticize. Should you select abortion, there is likely to be an emotional aftermath. Even great relief may be mingled with regret and sadness as you mourn the loss of the baby you wish you might have had.

On the other hand, prenatal diagnosis such as amniocentesis might offer assurance that the defect you feared was apparently not present in your unborn child. You would then be relieved of your fear and be able to experience the remainder of the pregnancy with enjoyment.

Alternate Routes to Parenthood

Adoption

A couple who are apprehensive about having another baby are

often consoled, "Never mind, you can adopt." Adoption may indeed be a wise solution, but it is not necessarily an easy one.

The availability of babies and children for adoption varies considerably in relation to other conditions in our society. For example, as safe and legal abortions become easier to obtain, fewer unwanted babies are likely to be born. Furthermore, an increasing number of babies born to unmarried parents are being reared by their parents. On the other hand, gradually widening acceptance of interracial families may increase the ease of adopting babies from minority groups within this nation as well as from abroad. Therefore, should you be considering adoption as an alternative, it would be most important to obtain current information from the staff of a child-welfare agency. (Adoptions are handled by both private and public agencies. In general, private agencies have more flexible adoption policies.)

There are many misconceptions about adoption practices. One worried young woman mistakenly believed that a couple would be considered eligible to adopt only if they owned their own home and could provide a separate bedroom for the adopted baby. Agencies do not necessarily seek wealthy homes, nor do they expect to find ideal parents. They do, however, seek parents who will be able to provide a standard of living above the poverty level and reasonably devoted care.

Should you decide to adopt, you are likely to be asked some of the questions raised in this chapter: after the needs of your afflicted child are met, will there be time, energy, interest, and affection available for an adopted child? Will you be able to accept an adopted child as a unique, individual personality, without asking him or her to stand in the footsteps of your ill child and to do what the ill child was unable to do? Since the adopted child was not the product of physical love between you and your spouse, might you feel that the child was not quite your own?

You may feel some discomfort, even resentment, that you are asked to think about and discuss such very personal matters. Interviews with an adoption agency staff member (often a trained social worker) may seem like an invasion of privacy; the visits to your home may seem like snooping. However, at present no better way is known of fulfilling the goals of the adoption agency: to determine which baby and which adoptive couple can best meet each other's needs.

Artificial Insemination

In this procedure, a small amount of semen obtained from a donor is inserted into the vagina of the woman by a physician. If this is done during the woman's fertile period — close to the time when an ovum is released from her ovary and travels across the fallopian tube to her uterus — it is likely that one of the millions of sperm contained in the semen will find its way into the ovum and conception will occur.

For some women, pregnancy is one of the most meaningful and satisfying experiences in life. Therefore, if a couple feels it necessary to avoid pregnancy because of the risk of having a child with an autosomal recessive disorder (one in which both partners carry the genetic trait), artificial insemination does offer a way in which the wife, at least, can experience biological parenthood. But if the disorder is a sex-linked condition carried by the female (such as hemophilia), artificial insemination is not the answer.

Furthermore, artificial insemination should be considered only if one can be sure that the donor does not also have the genetic trait that is of concern. Current information about this would have to be obtained from your family doctor, genetic counselor, or gynecologist. If it is possible to screen a donor for this trait, then the most significant question for a couple to consider is this: will artificial insemination affect the intimate bond between man and wife? A husband may feel that his wife has somehow been unfaithful to him through becoming impregnated by another man's sperm — it is as though there had been an adulterous interference in their intimate relationship. He may feel inadequate because his sperm were "less desirable" for his wife than those of another man. His wife, in turn, may feel guilt because she has participated in this somehow "unfaithful" act, or she may feel that her husband's special value to her is diminished.

Such feelings are not always present, and they can sometimes be openly shared between a couple, examined, and dispelled. However, the relationship between parents of a child with a serious disorder is already subject to strain from the worries arising from the illness. Artificial insemination can impose further strain, and perhaps should not be chosen unless the couple has deep confidence in the strength of their marital bonds.

Sources of Help

Effective Teamwork with the Doctor

During the time that your child is afflicted with his disorder, his doctor will be one of the most significant figures in your lives. There are many things that can be done to foster effective teamwork between doctor and family. Perhaps first among these is to establish which doctor will have primary responsibility for your child's care.

The Physician with Primary Responsibility

You may customarily seek medical care from a general practitioner or pediatrician in your community. When your child develops an unusual or dangerous illness, however, you (and the doctor) may urgently seek a specialist who knows about the most powerful drugs, the newest surgical methods, and the promise of research to combat the particular illness. Such a specialist is sometimes found in private practice, perhaps working with a group of associates. If your child's disorder is one that requires sophisticated laboratory tests and complex therapeutic equipment, the specialist is more likely to be found in a medical center, working with numerous "satellites" — associates, fellows, resident physicians and interns, and medical students. Your family doctor or pediatrician may arrange for the specialist to see your child in consultation only, and then continue as the responsible physician himself. Alternately, your child may become the private patient of the specialist or a staff patient in his section or department, such as the chest service, cardiac service, hematology service. Your child may also be referred to other sections, perhaps the chemotherapy section or the radiology department, for treatment. Tests may be done in the pulmonary physiology section or in the cardiac catheterization laboratory. This array of professions and specialized services can seem strange and frightening. It may help you to avoid moments of helpless confusion, anxiety, disappointment, and anger if, at the outset, you seek answers to the following questions:

1. Which doctor will have primary and continuing responsibility in making decisions about your child's medical care?

2. Which doctor will have primary and continuing responsibility for giving you medical information about your child?
3. Is this doctor willing to have occasional private conferences with you (not in the presence of your child) to review your questions, hopes, and fears?
4. Will this doctor assume responsibility for your child's total medical care (including immunizations and routine matters, such as upset stomachs and colds, eating habits, toilet habits, sleeping patterns, and physical activity)? Or will he limit his responsibility to management of the illness, and encourage you to consult your family doctor or pediatrician about other aspects of the child's health and development?
5. How can he be reached in person? By phone? May he be called at home?*
6. At what hours can he be reached in person? By phone?
7. If he is not available, and you are urgently concerned about your child, whom should you call?
8. For what reasons should he be called — for example, what symptoms or changes in your child's appearance should be reported to him?

Reaching an accord with the doctor about when he should be called may be a slow and clumsy process in your developing partnership to help your child. The doctor needs to learn your skill as an observer, your accuracy as a reporter, and your characteristic level of worry. You need to learn to distinguish chronic symptoms from those that signify a worrisome change or need for medical attention. You need to learn to trust your own observations and judgments. You need to become familiar with the doctor's expectations. The more forthright you can be about what you can and cannot cope with, the more likely you are to develop an effective rapport with your doctor. He needs to understand your needs.

Gathering Information

All of us, at times, shrink from seeking information that we fear will be disagreeable. The mother of a very ill child expressed this clearly in saying, "I don't ask questions. If the doctors have good news, they'll

---

*Do not overlook the corollary: how can *you* be reached? A busy doctor recently complained, with justifiable annoyance, that after receiving word that an anxious mother had phoned his office, he had made 14 attempts to return her call, each time getting the busy signal, before he was successful. Feeling panicky, she had called a sympathetic friend and talked for 75 minutes.

find me." Her attitude reflected the ancient belief that what you don't know can't hurt you. Understandable as is this belief, it is not usually helpful. Information can play a crucially important part in successful coping with a crisis such as your child's potentially serious disorder.

Information can help to relieve the powerful emotional responses parents commonly experience upon learning of their child's illness. For example, the sense of failure, the self-reproach, the guilt that most such parents feel is more readily dispelled if the parent is clearly informed that the child's illness was quite unrelated to anything the parents did, felt, or thought. The impulse to fight, the aggressive and angry feelings that may be aroused in parents can be constructively discharged if the parents learn of ways in which they can indeed fight for the child and against the illness. Apprehension can be relieved. First, as the parent finds out what he can do for his child, his sense of helplessness is reduced. Second, the dangers he imagines for his child may be considerably more fearful that those that exist in reality. This was shown in a study of 63 children with rheumatic fever and their parents. Parents of 38 of the children expected their children to have permanent heart weakness or damage; parents of 21 of the children expected their children to be permanently disabled and subject to continued restriction of activity. In fact, only three of these children were expected by their doctors to have any abnormality of the heart or to require restriction of activity. Therefore, it is clear that what you don't know can indeed hurt you. In fact, without a clear grasp of the realities of your child's illness, you cannot plan or act in a rational way on his behalf, your family's, or your own.

Parents of ill children are often very poorly informed. (In the rheumatic fever study, it was found that 78% of the parents had confused and incorrect ideas about their child's illness.) A basic reason for this is that physicians, as well as parents, sometimes fail to understand that becoming informed is a continuing process; it is not a happening. It is not rare for a busy specialist to plan only a single conference in which he explains to parents the cause, treatment, and outlook of their child's illness. At the conclusion of this conference, when he has transmitted the information he knows to be important, he may genuinely believe that the parents have been fully informed. Unfortunately, one session of explaining rarely, if ever, results in a worried, shocked, or grieved parent's becoming informed.

Many factors can interfere with an effective flow of information, and these factors make repetition essential. First, as has been pointed out in Chapter 1, parents (and all other human beings) need to protect themselves against painful realities, and to do so, they may deny, disbelieve, "switch off," "screen out," fail to hear. They can comprehend what the physician is telling them only little by little over a period of time. A wise and compassionate physician who takes care of children with blood diseases once remarked, "If you have to tell parents their child has leukemia, from the moment you mention that word you could be telling them that the sky is pink and they would never know what you are saying." Many parents can verify this: from the moment they heard the words *cystic fibrosis, cancer, heart disease,* or many others, they heard nothing more the doctor said in that interview. Unfortunately, a doctor may underestimate the degree to which worry and fear can interfere with parental understanding. This may be particularly true if a parent appears calm, seems to be listening attentively, nods at appropriate moments, asks a "sensible" question, or asks no questions at all. Therefore, it can be most important for a confused or uninformed parent to say to the doctor, "I was too upset to hear what you told me yesterday. Could we arrange time to go over it again?" It is likely that the doctor will appreciate your frankness, since it will help him know how to help you.

Difficulty in understanding the medical terms used by the doctor can interfere with information gathering. Medicine, like many other fields of special knowledge, has its own private language. This nomenclature, which fosters precise and efficient communication among physicians, becomes valued (along with the instruments of diagnosis and treatment) as an essential part of the professional expertise. Therefore, some physicians do feel a little more professional if they speak of the "bifurcation of the trachea" rather than of the "division of the air passage into two parts." Physicians in teaching hospitals who spend much time communicating with students and physicians-in-training, as well as with highly specialized professional colleagues, may readily overestimate a parent's knowledge of human biology; they may experience real difficulty in attempting to describe highly complex bodily functions with everyday language. They may forget that many laymen are unfamiliar even with such common terms as *congenital, cardiac,* and *seizure.*

Curiously, it is difficult indeed for parents to say, "I don't understand the words you are using, doctor." Perhaps the parent feels anxious to please the doctor (whose skills are so desperately needed for his child) or perhaps he fears that the doctor would be annoyed if he were told he is not understood and that more time for explanation is needed. The parent may feel that he would appear stupid, or at least not too intelligent, if he revealed his failure to understand. Furthermore, the parent may feel safer if the doctor uses a special language, because this offers assurance that the doctor is indeed an expert with special knowledge.

However, clear communication with the doctor is essential if you are to become informed about your child's illness. For this reason, it is most important to let him know that the terms he uses are strange to you, and to ask if he can explain in a simpler way. You might ask if he would be willing to send you a letter summarizing the explanation he has given you. You might also ask if there is other written material available for the layman.*

Parents are sometimes unsuccessful in gathering information because they have failed to prepare for a conference with the doctor. There is great value in spending a few quiet moments in advance of the conference thinking about what you and your family wish to learn from the doctor; it may be useful to make a few written notes to serve as reminders.

The circumstances under which the conference is held will very much influence the quality of communication. Too often, particularly in a busy medical center, the importance of privacy is overlooked by the staff. Parents find medical students, associate physicians, nurses and therapists present while they see the doctor, and are often troubled because discussion about the child's condition takes place around his examining table or bed. In attempting to balance his triple role as teacher of students, adviser of parents, and doctor of patients, the physician may at times overlook your continuing need for private communication. It may be necessary to let him know of this need, perhaps requesting a separate conference time for yourself.

Communication involves interaction of two personalities, not just of two minds. Therefore, a personality clash between parent and doctor can interfere significantly with information gathering. It was pointed out in Chapter 1 that an upsurge of angry feelings and aggressive impulses is experienced by many parents facing a threat to their child. Since one needs to feel angry at something or someone, it is not unusual for parents to feel angry at and critical, and mistrustful of their child's doctor, at least temporarily. Doctors, who have emotional needs like those of other people, react in varying ways according to their personalities. Some

---

*Pamphlets written for parents about a particular disorder can be a most helpful source of information. They are likely to be written in nontechnical language. They can be read at a time and in a place more relaxed than the doctor's office. They can be reviewed again and again without apology. They can be shown to relatives, friends, and baby-sitters. Should your child's doctor not have such pamphlets available, they may be procured through the voluntary health agencies concerned with particular illnesses (see Appendix).

share the compassionate understanding of one young physician caring for children with chest diseases: "Parents of sick children have to be angry at someone. I can absorb the anger." Another physician, however, may find his self-esteem shaken by the hostility of the parent of a child he is trying to help, and may respond with irritability or resentment.

In instances in which the clash arises from the parent's feeling of anguish and protest about his child's illness, anger toward the doctor often subsides as the parent comes to recognize the doctor's interest and concern. Occasionally, it does not; or a clash arising from personality differences continues unabated. In such instances, it is wise to be as frank as possible: "Doctor, I respect your experience and knowledge, but we seem to rub each other the wrong way all the time." This may lead either to more understanding and successful partnership between parent and doctor or to a mutual decision that it would be best for one of his associates to be available for your questions.

Information is gained only in part from the words the physician uses, the facts he helps you to understand. You will seek, urgently at times, information about his feelings and attitudes about your child's illness. Does he feel worried or confident? Is he discouraged or hopeful? You will search his facial expression, his tone of voice, even the way he moves about and holds his body for clues; and you may readily reach incorrect conclusions from what you observe. The doctor may appear discouraged because another patient is not doing well; he may appear defeated because he has been up all night dealing with an emergency; he may appear irritable because an important laboratory test was spoiled by a technician's carelessness. The only way to clarify whether your impression of his feelings about your child is correct is by putting it into words: "Doctor, you seem discouraged about Johnny. Am I right?" He may reply, "I am discouraged today, but it has nothing to do with Johnny."

Traditionally, communication about a child's health needs and problems takes place between his mother and the doctor. Only rarely is his father included. In the case of long-term or serious illness, such an arrangement imposes a heavy burden of responsibility on the mother. Not only must she inform herself about the child's needs, she must also communicate to the doctor the questions and concerns of her husband and family and convey the information the doctor imparts back to them. If there are any difficulties in her own relationship with the doctor, she may feel little confidence in bringing her hopes, fears, and needs to his attention without her husband's support. Therefore, it is most important that parents take the initiative in requesting opportunities to see the doctor together. A father can usually arrange time off from work for this purpose without loss of pay. If not, many doctors are willing to arrange an occasional evening appointment.

As has been pointed out, many things can interfere with successful information gathering: your anxiety and need to "switch off," difficulty understanding medical terms, failure to prepare for a conference, lack of privacy, a personality clash, misinterpretation of nonverbal clues, failure of both parents to participate. Therefore, it is essential to offer the physician some feedback on the information he has given. From time to time, it is most helpful to say, "Doctor, so far this is my understanding of what you have been telling me. Am I understanding you correctly?" This allows for review of the information, repetition as necessary, and for correction of any confused or mistaken ideas. To form a partnership with a physician that can be helpful for your child and family, you, as well as he, must take active responsibility for successful communication.

Crucial Questions

What Made My Child Get Sick?

All parents ask this question — urgently. Encouraged from childhood to think in terms of cause-effect relationships, they find it frightening and unacceptable to view a potentially serious illness as a chance event.

Few parents actually seek detailed information about the disordered physiological functions that have resulted in the illness. Rather, there are two pressing concerns: "Was I responsible for the illness?" "Could it happen to others in the family?" Talking these two questions over realistically with the doctor can help to dispel worry.

Jerry's mother (Chapter 1) feared that she had been responsible for his encephalitis. Her reasoning went thus: she had given Jerry permission to go fishing when he had the sniffles; he had fallen in the water and become soaked; the soaking must have made his sniffles develop into the severe illness which affected his brain; therefore, her permission to go fishing had led to his illness, and she was to blame. The doctor was able to point out: Jerry's infection was caused by a virus transmitted by a mosquito; such infections are not caused by soaking or chilling; the sniffles were probably a sign that the infection was already developing, and the result would have been the same whether or not Jerry went fishing; there is no way a child can be protected from all risk of infection.

Priscilla's mother (page 5) thought she had heard that leukemia can be brought on by emotional upsets. She feared that the constant quarrels between her husband and her might have been responsible for Priscilla's illness. The doctor was able to say: "It's hard for parents when we don't yet know the exact cause of a disease. However, leukemia develops in upset homes and happy homes, in rich homes and poor homes — all children experience some emotional stress in the course of growing up, and only a very few develop leukemia. I don't believe that your marital problems had anything to do with Priscilla's becoming sick."

The doctor who took care of Dave and Dorothy's son (page 6) explained that the baby's development had gone awry during the early months in the womb; his heart defect was one of nature's accidents, as surely as is a deformed tree in a forest, or a stunted flower in the garden, or a kitten born with six toes. Dave and Dorothy's premarital sexual relationship had no influence whatsoever on the baby's development. Dave's anguish arose from his innermost doubts about his worth as a human being; his torment could best be relieved in personal counseling.

In these instances of an *infectious* illness, an *acquired* illness of unknown cause, and a *congenital* illness from faulty intrauterine development, there was no reason — in reality — to believe that the parents were to blame or that others in the family would be afflicted. However, many of the disorders of concern to readers of this book are inherited — genetically transmitted. Since parents of children with genetically transmitted illnesses often find the question of their responsibility and the vulnerability of other family members particularly complex and troublesome, these disorders are discussed separately (pages 205-211).

What about the Treatment?

Most of the disorders of concern to readers of this book are not, *today*, curable. Progressively, however, medical science offers more effective treatment to slow the course or offset the effects of such disorders. A significant part of the treatment must usually be carried out at home.

Why Should You Do the Treatment?   At first, such a question sounds absurd. However, physicians have become gravely concerned about the number of patients and families who fail to comply with medical advice. Therefore, it is important to consider why it is desirable for you to carry out recommended treatment.

Foremost, the treatment helps your child physically — it helps to make him feel better and to keep him feeling better. Second, the treatment helps your child psychologically; it communicates that you care about him, that you value his well-being enough to persist and insist (even if he resists). It communicates that his situation is not hopeless, that there are things to be done for him. Third, compliance safeguards your own self-esteem. If you fail to carry out treatment, you can scarcely avoid some feelings of guilt and shame. If your child should become worse, or even die, your self-reproach could become unbearable.

What Helps You Comply? Research has been done to learn what factors influence people most strongly to follow medical advice. An acceptance that the treatment program is worthwhile, even crucial, has been identified as one important factor. Such acceptance can be strengthened if parents seek the answers to the questions: Why, how, when and where should treatment be done?

The question of *why* treatment is done is one of continuous importance to both you and your child, since understanding it can motivate you both to carry out the treatment. You may seek a very simple explanation or a highly sophisticated one. In either case, it is essential to learn enough so that you can feel confident that the treatment makes good sense. It is essential to know if treatment is expected to prevent or to control or to cure certain manifestations or complications of the illness.

The *how* of treatment concerns the nature of your child's medical program: regulation of his diet; giving medicine in the form of syrups, pills, ointments, inhalants, injections; manipulating his body through massage, exercise or postural drainage; supporting his body with braces or a wheelchair.

The program may at first seem overwhelming. However, your sense of confidence can be increased if you ask for: (1) clear, written instructions from the doctor, including diagrams if needed (for example, to show where an injection should be given, or how the body should be positioned for physical therapy); and (2) personal demonstrations by the professional staff, either in the medical center or in your home community. Long before you can consider pushing a needle into your child's skin, you will need practice sessions supervised by a registered nurse. A physical therapist can first show you how to do massage or postural drainage, and then watch you do it. A dietitian can tell you how to make a medicine palatable; how to prepare a special diet. Such professionals are eager to help, but you should make known your need.

The *how* also concerns the age and development of your child. Does he yet, for example, have enough control over his tongue and throat movements so that he can swallow a pill? Will he understand that the chest clapping before postural drainage is treatment, or will he view it as a kind of spanking? Does he have the skill, judgment, and motivation to give his own injections? Many such questions have already been considered in this book. They are important matters to discuss with a pediatrician well grounded in child development, as well as with nurses, dietitians, and physiotherapists experienced with children.

The *when* of treatment must take into account its medical effectiveness. For example, certain medications should be given at certain intervals of time and in certain relationships to meals. Others can be given on a more flexible basis according to your judgment about your child's condition (confidence in such judgment develops slowly in most parents). The *when* should also take into account your child's routine. You might, for example, choose to do physiotherapy as he watches his favorite TV cartoons. You might try to avoid interrupting a pleasurable play session with his friends or choosing a time of day when he is almost always cranky. The *when* must also take into consideration the needs of others — the times when other family members need your special attention, the time of day that is your low period.

The *where* of home treatment is determined chiefly by the arrangement of your home and by your personal preferences. If treatment lasts more than a few moments, it can be helpful to your mood if you choose a bright and cheerful room, and perhaps play some lighthearted music or listen to an amusing radio or TV program.

If treatment requires bedrest, it is worthwhile to consider how your child's room can be made as appealing as possible. If the room does not get much light, perhaps the walls might be painted pale yellow. (If moisture is needed in the room, mildew-resistant paint should be selected.) The ceiling — which he will see so often — might be decorated with interesting decals, or you might encourage friends and relatives who ask about gifts to pool their resources for a projection box that casts changing patterns and rhythms of colored light across the ceiling. You might hang, in turn, a variety of mobiles where they will respond to moving air currents and arrange a changing exhibition of posters or the child's art work on the walls.*

The child may feel safer if he is in communication with others in the family. If his own phone extension or an intercom is beyond your means, he might have a small cowbell by his bed. A signal system could be arranged to communicate: "lonely — need company"; "help needed"; "feeling sick."

If your child's stools have an especially foul odor, or if he vomits frequently, provision will be needed for adequate ventilation of the bathroom by window or exhaust fan. A time-honored method of dispelling odor is by burning a wooden match.

If food is served in bed, keep in mind the patient's difficulty drinking out of an ordinary cup or glass without having the liquid dribble

---

*Remember that freezer tape, unlike cellophane tapes, leaves no gummy residue on the paint.

down his chin. A small pitcher or teapot with a long spout makes an excellent utensil for in-bed drinking. A plastic infant cup with lid and
spout does also, if it does not offend the patient's dignity.

Why Might You Fail to Comply?   Parents sometimes give up (or
never start) treating their child because he doesn't really seem sick. If he
is in an early stage of an illness, has a mild case, or is in a period of remission (of temporary improvement), he may have few symptoms. It is
natural to try to think of him as healthy, and to encourage him to view
himself as healthy. Carrying out treatment can be a distressing reminder
of his disorder, and it is understandable that parents might prefer to
avoid it. Furthermore, when a child does not appear sick, parents may
fail to carry out treatment because they do not understand its preventive
purpose. For example, the long-term penicillin treatments for children
who have had rheumatic fever and the postural drainage for children
with cystic fibrosis are largely preventive measures. It is understandable
that parents might hope that the child would get along just as well
without the treatment.

Parents sometimes give up treatment because the child is in a particularly negative phase of development, and treatment may provoke
disagreeable fights between the protesting child and the insisting parent.
Parents may also give up treatment because they feel discouraged, even
hopeless, about the child's future.

Feelings of shame may make it very difficult for such parents to
reveal their noncompliance to the doctor. It may be helpful to explore
the problem first with another professional, such as a trained social
worker. When the reasons for the difficulty with treatment are understood, then it may be possible to work out, with the doctor, a compromise solution that is appropriate for parent and child.

Is There Hope?

No question can be more desperately important to you than this
one. It is a question that many well-meaning people may try to answer —
whether or not they are qualified, whether or not you have asked them.
Friends and relatives, parents of similarly affected children, doctors and
nurses all may offer conflicting opinions and make contradictory predictions. You may find yourself actively collecting such opinions, perhaps
from a lingering sense of disbelief that the illness is real, perhaps because
you still long to prove that the doctor is wrong. However, collecting
opinions can scarcely give you genuine help, since in every affected child
the course of an illness is individual. The only person who can reliably

tell you the outlook for your child is the doctor who has primary responsibility for his care.

What Are the Odds?   You need to know whether or not it is realistic to feel hopeful about your child. You may find yourself asking, "What are his chances?" "What are the odds?" Even if you have not asked, the doctor may talk to you in these terms, perhaps showing you graphs and charts concerned with the disorder. He may do this because he, too, cares about your child, and it is less sorrowful to talk about statistics than about one little blue-eyed boy named Billy. He may do this because otherwise he will need to say, "I don't know," and this sometimes makes doctors (and everyone else) feel helpless.

Some parents feel most comfortable if information can be expressed in charts and diagrams. Rarely is it genuinely helpful for you to know the statistical odds. The odds are computed on the basis of large numbers of cases. There is no way to know which of those many cases might be like your own child — which statistic is named Billy?

The odds have been computed on the basis of past knowledge about the disorder and its treatment. Is there any reason to believe the odds will be the same tomorrow?

Parents of children with extended illness are sometimes asked to accommodate to an agonizing succession of predictions: "The chances are ___% that your child will reach school age." "The chances are ___% that your child will become a teenager." "The chances are ___% that your child will survive adolescence." As more and more is learned about the disorder and its management, the earlier prediction becomes invalid and a new one is set forth, each prediction arousing new hope, new despair, or utter bewilderment ("What can I believe?"). It is therefore essential to keep in mind that a prediction about your child's future is based only on the medical knowledge that exists today.

What about Research?

Seven years ago, a slender, dainty nine-year-old blonde girl was hospitalized in a children's clinical research center.* Two years before, she had been found to have a rare, highly malignant tumor that no child had been known to survive. She had undergone extensive surgery to remove the original tumor and others that had developed later. As a last hope, she was brought to the center for a trial of a newly developed anticancer drug. Today, that girl is a vibrant, active high-school student.

Medicine has made dramatic, even unbelievable advances in the

---

*Such centers have been developed in selected medical centers throughout the nation with funds disbursed through the National Institutes of Health, an agency within the Department of Health, Education, and Welfare.

last quarter century. As one patient declared, "If it weren't for research, things would be way back where they were a long time ago." There are new methods to make precise diagnoses, new surgical techniques to repair or replace diseased body parts, new machines to assist the body in carrying out its vital functions, new understanding of the body's responses to germs, new drugs to offset the ravages of disease. These advances have been the result of clinical research — the careful, repeated observation of the effects that result from certain known causes. For families of ill or disabled children and for the children themselves, research is, appropriately, a major source of hope.

In the stormy period when you first struggle to face your child's disorder, you may feel a frantic need to know about research. This need renders you vulnerable since false hope can easily be aroused by newspaper and magazine accounts of remarkable cures and by the reports of friends, neighbors, and relatives who have heard of apparent miracles. You are vulnerable because such reports, published for their dramatic news value (newspapers, after all, must be sold), are often premature. That is, they are often based on early impressions about a cause-effect relationship that have not been confirmed through careful, repeated observations. You are vulnerable because you have no basis for judging whether the research workers are competent, whether the research was well planned and carried out, whether the results might have occurred only by chance. You cannot judge whether a new medicine has been sufficiently tested to have been proven safe. The only way to know whether such reports hold promise for your child is by discussing them with the doctor, preferably bringing to him the article you have seen.

Parents sometimes wonder how their child's doctor can stay up to date about research findings. There are several ways in which this is done. It is likely that he receives one or more publications that contain abstracts — brief summaries — of the most significant recent articles that have been published in a wide variety of medical journals. These may include reports of completed research as well as notations concerning research that is in progress.

If the doctor is on the staff of a medical center, he will be in repeated, perhaps daily, contact with other specialists, and, even over a morning cup of coffee or walking down the stairs, may be gaining information helpful to your child. If he is in private practice, he may attend seminars and conferences in the nearest medical center,* and periodic

*Under the leadership of the Regional Medical Programs Services (an agency of the Department of Health, Education, and Welfare), medical schools and centers throughout the country are being encouraged to share the wealth of their knowledge, experience, and facilities with private physicians and community hospitals in a systematic way.

medical meetings in other cities. In these ways, he will learn of research even before it is reported in the medical journals; and he may choose to contact the scientist or doctor doing a particular piece of research if he feels it could hold promise for your child.

Should Your Child Participate in Research?   Research can be a source of hope. Parents may, in fact, be as fervent as one parent who declared, "Growth hormone is my religion right now." Research can also arouse fear and worry in the parent whose own child is to become a research patient. Some parents worry that, "out of scientific curiosity," the doctors might do more tests than are necessary for the child's needs. Some fear that the research might harm the child rather than help him.

Mistrust and fear of research with human subjects has been an aftermath of the inhuman atrocities performed in the name of research by Nazi scientists and physicians. These ghastly episodes did, however, result in an earnest and conscientious consideration being given to safeguarding the dignity and welfare of research subjects. Guidelines intended to insure that research would be carried out in a humane and ethical manner were set forth by the World Medical Organization in a document known as the Declaration of Helsinki.*

Much of the clinical research (research in which human patients are the subjects) carried out in the United States in recent years has been supported by federal funds administered by the National Institutes of Health (NIH). This agency wisely made it a condition that each medical center receiving NIH research funds should supervise all research with human subjects carried out by its physicians and scientists.† In most centers such supervision is carried out by a clinical investigation committee, whose membership ideally includes persons able to evaluate the ethical, legal, psychological, and scientific aspects of a particular study. A detailed description of each proposed research project is studied by such a committee, which directs its concern toward the welfare of the patient as well as toward the scientific merit of the research.

Physicians in the United States have traditionally disliked and resisted regulation. For this reason — perhaps chiefly to assert his independence — an occasional physician in a medical center may bypass such a committee. If you would find such reassurance helpful, it would not be inappropriate to ask your child's doctor whether a particular research program has been approved by a clinical investigation committee.

*British Medical Journal 2(1964): 177.
†New guidelines are currently being drawn up by the Department of Health, Education, and Welfare.

One of the most important principles set forth in the Declaration of Helsinki, and widely accepted since, is that no research with human subjects should be carried out without the informed consent of the subject. In the case of research with children, the informed consent of the parent or legal guardian is essential. Therefore, if it is suggested that your child participate in a clinical research project or that a research drug be tried for his disorder, it is reasonable to seek answers to the following kinds of questions:

1. What is the purpose of the research? In what ways could this research benefit your child? Can immediate benefit for your child be expected, or is future benefit the only possibility? Is there an alternative way of helping your child?
2. Where will the studies be done? Will the research necessitate overnight hospitalization, daytime hospitalization? For how many days? Can the studies or tests be done in the doctor's office or at home? Will your child be admitted to a special research unit or to a regular children's division?
3. What procedures will be included? What will your child undergo in the way of procedures such as x-rays, stool and urine collections, injections, or intravenous infusions? Many parents find it helpful to ask for a written, day-by-day plan so that they can prepare themselves as well as their child for the procedures.
4. What are the risks? Are there physical risks from any of the procedures to be carried out? Are there risks from medications to be given, especially unpleasant or possibly harmful side effects? Are there emotional risks for the child, such as from anxiety related to separation from the family or from procedures that could be intensely distressing or frightening to him?
5. How can the risks be minimized? It is most likely that the physician conducting the research (who may or may not be the doctor with primary responsibility for your child's care) will have taken every possible precaution against physical risk. He may, however, have given little consideration to emotional risk.* Therefore, you may need to take some initiative in bringing up this topic. You may also find it helpful to ask for a conference with the head nurse or social worker associated with the research center or ward if your child is to be hospitalized. In such a conference, held *before* admission, plans can be

---

*In a series of interviews with parents prior to the admission of their children to a children's clinical research center, the author found that in almost all instances the physicians had conscientiously and frankly discussed physical risk with the parents before asking them to give consent, but had rarely considered emotional risk.

made to safeguard your child's emotional well-being and the well-being of your family. (The specific hazards of hospitalization at different periods of a child's development have been discussed in Chapters 3-6).

Is the Timing of the Admission Elective? In some cases, it is urgent that a trial of a research drug be started as soon as possible. In other instances, it is appropriate to be flexible about planning the admission. If your doctor believes that flexiblity is permissible, you may wish to time the admission in relation to other family events and needs. Perhaps, for example, you will be able to arrange for household help; or one parent will arrange time off from work so that the other parent will be able to spend considerable time with the child in the hospital.

If possible (unless it is to be an emergency admission), explore all the above questions with your child's doctor in a special conference arranged in advance of the admission. Although you may have to press for such a conference,* almost all parents find it extremely helpful in relieving their own anxieties about research and in informing themselves about what they and their child can expect. It is much more useful to talk out your fears and uncertainties with the doctor than — because you are apprehensive and confused — to seek multiple opinions from unqualified sources. Only if you take responsibility for informing yourself, can you give informed consent on behalf of your child.

Should Your Child Give Consent? Serious consideration is currently being given to the question of whether or not school-age children should themselves be expected to give consent before participating in clinical research. This question is especially crucial with respect to children participating in research that is not expected to benefit them directly (such research is designed to increase medical understanding of a particular physiological process or disease entity and later to benefit other children). Such a situation would rarely arise for readers of this book, since few parents of children with impaired health would themselves agree to research if it was expected to impose further stress upon the child without offering any hope of benefit.

However, the question of the child's consent also applies in instances when it is hoped that the research procedures or medication will control or cure the child's own illness. In a situation of this nature, the important consideration is whether the child is intellectually capable and emotionally free to give meaningful consent.

---

*Physicians in a modern medical center are subject to many pressures. In addition to the urgent task of helping ill people recover, there may be teaching responsibilities and an expectation that the physician will carry out research and publish his work in scientific journals. Therefore, the needs of families for reassuring and informative communication are sometimes overlooked unless brought to the physician's attention.

It seems doubtful that this would be the case with many children before adolescence. Although school-age children are able to understand cause-effect relationships concerning sensations or events they directly observe or experience,* only gradually do they become intellectually able to grasp abstract ideas beyond the realm of their experience. Research is an abstract and complex idea that many adults have difficulty understanding. A child can scarcely make a meaningful judgment about an idea he cannot comprehend. Therefore, few pre-adolescent children could be considered intellectually capable of giving informed consent.

Furthermore, most children trust the adults responsible for their care, especially their parents and doctors, to safeguard their well-being. In addition, their need for the approval of these significant adults is deep and intense. For both these reasons, it is doubtful that most children are emotionally free to refuse a research procedure the adults recommend. If a child is not emotionally free to refuse, his consent is meaningless.

Even in adolescence, when the young person may be intellectually capable of understanding the idea of research, his comprehension may be clouded by fear. Furthermore, the adolescent characteristically has contradictory thoughts and conflicting emotions. These tendencies were recognized by two wise parents who remarked, "If we accept her refusal of the research now, she may reproach us bitterly later on and say, 'Why didn't you make me do it?' " Therefore, although it may be appropriate for the adolescent to take part in considering whether or not he should participate in the research, it could be unwise to base the decision on his refusal or consent.

When the adolescent is involved in making a decision about a procedure or medication that might entail serious risk, he is almost certain to need considerable help in sorting out and understanding his thoughts and feelings. Such help is most likely to be obtained from a person who is expert at communicating with teenagers — often a child psychiatrist or a specialist in adolescent medicine.

Preparing Your Child. Although it is doubtful that many children or adolescents are fully capable of giving free and informed consent, children of all ages need and have a right to careful preparation for the research experience, just as they do for hospitalization† or any other medical experience. Since an aura of mystery and magic often surrounds medical research, it is wise to make a particular effort to insure that the child's expectations are realistic, even while protecting his sense of hope.

*Chapter 4.

†Discussions of the theories of illness formed by the developing child are found in Chapters 4 and 5.

David, age 9, was hospitalized for a series of complex studies to determine whether a hormone deficiency was responsible for his abnormally small size. Although he endured the procedures with no more than appropriate protest and worry, after his return home he became despondent. He had no appetite, slept badly, and refused to attend school. His sympathetic father was able to learn that David had believed that the fluid in the intravenous infusions involved in the tests had been magical growth hormone. He had imagined that during his hospital stay he would grow and Grow and GROW.

One way to find out if your child's expectations of research are at least moderately realistic is to ask him, "If you were explaining the reason for the tests (or the medicine) to your best friend, what would you tell him?" You might also ask, "How do you suppose you'll be feeling when the tests (or the medicine) are finished?"

If the research does not produce the results you and your child have hoped for, each of you will doubtless feel a tremendous letdown — disappointment, sadness, and anger. One child furiously, but understandably, declared, "Dr. A. doesn't know anything. He was just using me for a pincushion." This child's medication had not resulted in a change in his condition.

It is wise, also, to be prepared for the possibility that the research effort will succeed. Although it would be a joy to have your child's condition improve markedly, it is wise to remember that if he does change, other people will expect more of him. He may be very much concerned about whether he will be able to measure up — to be fully adequate. He will need your support, not only in understanding his worry, but also in helping him to "hang loose," to take it one day at a time, during the period of improvement and readjustment.

What If My Child Should Die?

Agonizing as the question is, parents do at moments wonder, "What if things go badly — what if my child has a setback? What if he should die? What would it be like for him? Would the end be swift or prolonged? Would he be aware or would he slip into a coma? Would there be pain?"

Parents have found that it may be difficult indeed to gather such information. Their child's doctor may respond to such questions with an attempt to comfort: "Let's not think about that right now. Try to put it out of your mind." Unfortunately, there is no eject button for worrisome thoughts. You may need to say, "Doctor, it would be helpful to have such information; it would make us feel stronger to be a little bit prepared." It is likely, then, that he will be able to explain some of the things medicine can offer to ease pain and allow death to occur as easily and gently as possible for the child.

This may also be an appropriate time for you and the doctor to discuss your respective attitudes about heroic measures to extend life as long as possible or about some of the dramatic but still unreliable new techniques, such as organ transplants. Although it is the doctor's responsibility to recommend whatever treatment he believes appropriate, it may be helpful to him to know your beliefs and feelings about the more extreme measures.

Although after a prolonged illness the ending may offer some feeling of relief, there is no way, no way at all, that your child's death can be easy or gentle for you. You are likely to experience again the intense anguish aroused at the time of diagnosis* — the sorrow, the self-reproach, the anger, the apprehension. Your sleep may be disturbed by sad and frightening dreams; during the daytime you may feel exhausted, in emotional disarray, unable to get your head together. Although you may wonder if you are losing your mind, going crazy, what you are experiencing is profound grief, grief that affects almost every aspect of your physical, emotional, and mental functioning.

There will be people who wish to help — doctors, nurses, clergymen, social workers, friends, neighbors, relatives. Although none can take away your grief — much as they may wish to — they can help you to endure it until the passing of time softens it and the beckonings of those who need you again engage your mind and your heart.

How Will It Be Afterward?

It may be many months, or only a few weeks, before the harsh intensity of your grief begins to soften. There is no length of time you should grieve, no special way you should feel or behave. Your mourning will be influenced by many things, such as the nature and length of your child's illness, his age and temperament, your relationship with him, your relationships with other family members, your religious beliefs. If the final stage of your child's illness was a long one, or if he had come again and again to the brink of death, your sorrow may indeed be mingled with relief that his suffering has ended.

Painful as it is to return again to the hospital or doctor's office, many parents find it valuable to plan a follow-up conference with the doctor. The visit can help to dispel your feeling of unreality about the end — your disbelief that the child has actually died. A review of the

*Chapter 1.

final stages of the illness can answer questions that have arisen in your mind. It can also reassure you that you and the medical team gave your child the best possible care. It may also be helpful to see the staff member — nurse, chaplain or social worker — who offered the greatest support and solace. Such a person may be able to help you sort out the tangled web of your emotions.

The pattern of your daily life may have been organized around visiting your child in the hospital during his final illness. Even before that became necessary, his home treatment program probably affected your entire family. If the ill child needed attention in the morning, for example, his brothers and sisters may have needed to become independent in gathering their clothes, dressing, preparing their breakfasts, fixing their lunches, and departing for the bus. When the ill child is gone, there are likely to be huge empty spaces — not only emotional ones, but gaps in the household routine. The parent who had been most involved with the child's care is likely to feel unneeded, lost. How strange, in the morning, to sit with a cup of coffee watching the family bustling around you, no one expecting anything of you, almost behaving as though it didn't matter that you were there.

Your family will not easily be able to change their patterns of response or their routines. In fact, it may be more helpful for them if they don't immediately try. Therefore, you may need to look elsewhere to find the sense of significance — the awareness that your life does have meaning — which will gradually fill in the bleak emptiness. You may find it meaningful to volunteer some time to a school or library, to study a new language, to repaint your kitchen, or to play tennis. What you do is less important than that you do something you believe to be worthwhile.

Healing takes place slowly. For some time, your emotional wound is likely to be reopened again and again. The first time you pass your child's school or see his playmates, the first Christmas or Chanukah without him, the first family trip you plan, his birthday — again and again and again you will remember him; again and again and again your tears will flow. But gradually, imperceptibly, they will feel less like harsh, stinging sleet and more like a gentle spring rain.

Your spouse and your other children will reopen the wound as they themselves grieve. A preschool child, because he cannot yet grasp the idea of permanence, will ask over and over, "When is Paulie coming home?" Older brothers and sisters may try in various ways to deny or undo the loss. Some have tried desperately to regain contact with the dead one through extrasensory perception or a séance. Whatever their ages, they will need help (as described in Chapter 2): information to help them understand what has happened; explanations about your mood and probably altered behavior; permission to express their feelings openly and in their own fashion (if you find this unbearable, encourage them to contact a trusted friend, relative, teacher, clergyman, counselor, or doctor); reassurance about their own health and assurance that they were not to blame for what happened.

Inherited Illness and Genetic Counseling

It is difficult for most parents to gain a clear understanding of inherited, or genetically transmitted, illness. In part, this is because the speciality of human genetics has, like other scientific specialties, developed its own language. In seeking genetic information, the layman is quickly adrift in a sea of mysterious terms: *gametes* and *meiosis*, *haploid* and *diploid*, *alleles*, *homozygous*, *heterozygous* and *hemizygous*, *genotypes* and *phenotypes*, *locus* on the *chromosome*, *deoxyribonucleic acid*. A standard dictionary offers little assistance in clarifying their meanings; a recently edited high-school or college biology text may be more helpful, but only if it includes a precise glossary of terms. The following information is offered to help you understand the terms your child's doctor may use and to help you decide what questions to ask.

How Is Illness Inherited?

The human body is composed of millions of tiny units known as cells. Each cell is "programmed," or "instructed," to grow and develop in a particular way and to serve a special function in the body. The instructions come from within the core (the nucleus) of each cell.

Within the nucleus, there are long strands — or threadlike structures — *chromosomes*. These strands are composed of highly complex chemical matter (deoxyribonucleic acid on a framework of protein). Each segment of the chromosome is called a *gene*. It is the genes that, through their complex chemical influences, instruct the cell about its form and function.

Every normal human cell* includes 46 chromosomes arranged in 23 pairs. In a particular person, each cell contains the same 23 pairs; one member of each has been contributed at conception by the father's sperm cell, one member by the mother's ovum. It is entirely a matter of chance which chromosomes are received from which parent. There are

---

*Except the sex cells. In the course of their development, the male sperm and the female ovum undergo a process during which their 46 chromosomes are reduced to 23.

many trillions of possible chromosome combinations.

Twenty-two pairs of chromosomes are matched, and termed *autosomes*. The twenty-third pair includes the male—female sex chromosomes, which may or may not be matched (the sex *chromosomes* should not be confused with the sex *cells*, which have already been pointed out as the one type of normal cell having only 23 chromosomes). The matching chromosomes, or autosomes, are clusters of thousands of similarly matched genes. That is, each gene on a particular location of a chromosome has a partner in a corresponding location on the matching chromosome. Each matched pair of genes is concerned with the same genetic "business," such as eye color and whether hair will be curly or straight.

However, the instructions coming from the gene partners do not necessarily agree. Sometimes both partners will agree and both instruct, for example, "This baby is to have blue eyes." Pairs of genes that agree on their instructions are termed *homozygous* genes. Sometimes the instructions coming from each partner are different (one instructs "blue eyes" and one instructs "brown eyes"); such pairs of genes are termed *heterozygous*.

When a pair of heterozygous genes gives its mixed instructions, one of two results is possible: a compromise between the two different instructions occurs or the instructions of one partner have a stronger influence and dominate over the instructions from the other partner. In the latter case, the "stronger" gene is termed *dominant* and the "weaker" gene *recessive*.

Inherited illnesses are caused by defects in the cells that have been programmed by the genes. If an inherited illness has resulted from the instructions of a *dominant* gene, how might the inheritance pattern have worked? This can be illustrated by considering osteogenesis imperfecta. An individual might inherit a pair of genes concerned with the genetic characteristics of osteogenesis. Even if only one of the pair has the osteogenesis *trait* (in which case, it will instruct the cells to develop the osteogenesis defect) and the other member of the pair is normal, the gene with the osteogenesis trait will have a stronger influence and will dominate over the normal gene. This unfortunate individual will develop osteogenesis imperfecta.

Should this person, who has one osteogenesis gene (O) and a paired normal gene (N), mate with a person whose genes are normal (NN) insofar as osteogenesis is concerned, the outcome would appear thus (the genes are numbered only to indicate the possible ways in which each gene from the father might be paired with each gene from the mother in the offspring, each of whom will inherit a pair of genes concerned with osteogenesis):

1 2		3 4
O N		N N

1+3	2+3	1+4	2+4
O N	N N	O N	N N

Many persons believe, understandably, that such an outcome means that 50% of their children will have the illness and 50% will be normal. They believe, therefore, that if one afflicted child has already been born, it would be safe to have a second child since that child would surely be normal. Or it is believed that if there are two healthy children, the next two would have to be sick. If one were to count all the children born in the world to couples such as depicted in the chart above, it is probable that 50% of the children would be afflicted and 50% would be normal. However, in the individual family, the outcome can be quite different.

Each time such a couple has a child, there are two chances out of four that the child will inherit a gene having the osteogenesis trait; since this gene is dominant, the child will develop osteogenesis imperfecta. The odds of two out of four, or 50%-50%, will remain the same with each pregnancy, just as there is a 50-50 chance with every toss of a coin that either heads or tails will turn up.

In the case of disorders caused by dominant genes, it is likely that a family history of the disorder can be traced. That is, the illness has probably been seen in preceding generations, unless the disorder is extremely rare or only recently identified. In such cases, the illness may have been incorrectly diagnosed in earlier generations. On the other hand, genes do sometimes undergo mutation, becoming faulty for the first time. When this occurs, a disorder may appear in an individual whose family history is normal. He, then, may pass the disorder along to his offspring.

The majority of inherited disorders that would concern readers of this book — diseases such as cystic fibrosis, phenylketonuria, Tay-Sachs disease, Cooley's anemia, sickle cell anemia — are caused by recessive genes. If a recessive gene programmed for such a disorder is paired with a normal partner, the normal gene will dominate. Two such recessive genes must be paired together for the disorder to result (except in the case of sex-linked disorders, which are discussed later). Therefore, if a child has a disorder caused by recessive genes, the inheritance pattern will have operated thus:

C = Cystic fibrosis gene N = Normal gene

1 2   3 4
C N   *C N*

1+3   1+4   2+3   2+4
C C   *C N*   *N C*   *N N*

In such a case, neither parent has the illness; both parents have one normal gene and one cystic fibrosis gene and are therefore considered to "have the trait" (or to be *carriers**). A child can inherit such an illness only if both parents have the trait.

Such parents may have been entirely unaware that they carried the trait since there may be no known family history of the illness. For generations, those carrying the trait (*CN*) may have mated with normal individuals (*NN*), producing some children with the trait but none with the illness:

C N   *N N*

CN   *NN*   *CN*   *NN*

Among the children born to two parents both of whom carry such a trait, the chances are one in four that each child will inherit the illness (*CC*), two in four that he will inherit the trait (*CN*), and one in four that he will be normal (*NN*). Thus, in the individual family, the odds remain the same with each pregnancy. These odds are not influenced by what has already happened in that family; a particular family might have three successive children born with an inherited illness (such a tragedy has occurred in families known to the author) or 10 healthy children.

Most of the inherited defects and disorders are caused by genes located ·on the 22 matched pairs of chromosomes, the autosomes.

---

*It is unfortunate that this term is commonly used in discussing inheritance since it has also been used to refer to persons who harbor germs causing infectious illness, such as typhoid fever and hepatitis. Such persons may transmit illness to others, often because of careless personal hygiene. Therefore, in the minds of many people the term *carrier* suggests uncleanliness or outright dirtiness.

Therefore, the inheritance pattern is termed either *autosomal dominant* or *autosomal recessive*, depending on whether the disorder results from the influence of one dominant gene (overcoming the influence of its normal partner) or two recessive genes.

Some disorders are caused by the influence of genes located on the twenty-third pair of chromosomes, the sex chromosomes. Such disorders are called *sex-linked*. In the female, this twenty-third pair is composed of two "X" chromosomes. In the male, it is composed of one X and one Y. The Y chromosome is much smaller than the X and it contains fewer genes. As far as is known, its genetic activity is concerned almost exclusively with male sexual development. Therefore, sex-linked disorders are caused primarily by genes found on the X chromosomes, and usually by recessive genes. Color blindness and hemophilia A and B are examples of sex-linked, recessive disorders.

Although it is possible for the female to inherit two such recessive genes, one on each of her X chromosomes, this is not likely to occur. It is more usual for the female to be entirely normal and just carry the trait for a disorder such as hemophilia, having the recessive hemophilia gene on one X chromosome paired with a normal on the other X chromosome. Should she have a son, he might, by chance, inherit the X chromosome bearing the hemophilia gene rather than the X chromosome bearing the normal gene. This X chromosome would then be paired with the Y chromosome inherited from the father (which determined that he was a son rather than a daughter). There is no gene on the Y chromosome to counteract the hemophilia gene on the X chromosome. Therefore, even though only one recessive gene is present, this gene will act as though it is dominant and will produce the disorder in the male.

Genetic Counseling

Genetic *mis*information can be used as a weapon of attack, blame, and criticism within a troubled family. Genetic information can be relieving. It can be relieving to learn that one's genetic makeup has been determined not by one's thoughts, deeds, or character but by chance distribution of genes from among many trillions of possibilities. It can be relieving to realize that all human beings are believed to carry genes programmed to cause defects under certain conditions. To be human is to be imperfect. The carrier of an inherited disorder is different from others only if it is his misfortune that, by chance, a gene programmed to cause a defect was passed from him to his offspring and, again by chance, was perhaps paired with a similar gene from his mate. It can be relieving to understand the pattern of inheritance and to know whether other family members are likely to be affected.

Who can supply such information? Can this genetic counseling be carried out by a scientist with a Ph.D. in biology or by a social worker experienced in family counseling? Such persons do indeed have a contribution to make as members of the genetic counseling team. However, since the heart of the matter is a medical problem, the captain of the team should be the physician.

A physician is needed to make an exact diagnosis, since different forms of the same kind of disorder can have quite different causes. For example, a baby could be deaf at birth for many different reasons. He may have inherited one of several different kinds of genetic illness; his mother may have had an illness herself during her pregnancy that resulted in abnormal development of the unborn child; there may have been a particular complication during or right after delivery that caused the baby's condition.

A physician is needed to determine, sometimes through careful physical examinations and laboratory tests of relatives as well as from the medical history, whether the disorder is present in other family members. The findings will be evaluated by the physician, along with reports published in medical and scientific journals (to which the scientist with the Ph.D. in biology may have made a rich contribution). He will then be able to determine the probable inheritance pattern of a disorder in a particular family. If there is a risk that other children born in the family would have the same condition, the physician is needed to provide accurate medical information about family planning: contraception, sterilization, amniocentesis, abortion, artificial insemination.

Although such careful identification of an inherited disorder and informing the family about the pattern of inheritance is commonly referred to as *genetic counseling*, *genetic education* might be a more appropriate term. Families need not only information but also help in coming to terms with that information, and it is this help counseling should provide.

It is natural for parents whose children inherit a defect to feel regret and sadness. When the defect is mild and common, such as near-sightedness, the regret is probably mild and temporary. When the defect is serious, causing an extended illness, for example, the regret may be intense. Parents may feel guilty also — as though they have wronged their child. They may have feelings of shame, unworthiness, inadequacy, even feelings of being tainted and unclean. When such feelings are intense and persistent, one of the most useful things such troubled parents can do for their child and for themselves is to seek family counseling. A professional family counselor is trained to help parents explore, vent, and resolve their feelings and attitudes about carrying a genetic defect. A counselor is trained to help them understand its influence on their relationship, as well as to help them consider their attitudes about alternative methods of family planning.

An occasional geneticist may be well qualified to carry out such counseling. More usually a mental health professional is needed. A social worker associated with the genetics service may be able to offer such help or to arrange for it elsewhere.

Personal Counseling and Psychotherapy

The challenge of coping, and helping your child cope, effectively with extended illness is immense. Yet, curiously, it has often been observed that parents fail to make full use of the helping resources available to them. Many are unaware that such resources exist.

In part, this may be because medical care in the United States has become increasingly specialized. The patient with a complex disorder — and his family — tends to become locked into a medical service system in which the emphasis is on the disease rather than on the total patient. At the center of the system is the physician, who may be quite sensitive or quite insensitive to the patient's emotional, social, and spiritual needs. Therefore, even if there is a multi-discipline team (with professionals from varying backgrounds, such as nurses, social workers, psychologists, clergymen) within the medical facility, the physician may fail to perceive the need to refer his patient to such professionals.

On the other hand, sick people and their families tend to direct almost magical expectations toward their physicians. Because of their complex knowledge, their awesome skills and the apparent miracles that modern medicine has wrought — because, in fact, they do often exert life-and-death power — doctors are regarded as all-knowing and all-powerful.

Parents may fail to realize that only a rare physician can be at once a wise diagnostician and learned therapist, a calm and compassionate counselor, a brilliant research scientist. More usually, a physician is not all things to all men — he cannot fill with equal skill all the roles that are assigned to him.

It is usually realistic, therefore, not to expect the child's doctor to meet all of your child's needs (or yours). It is wise to seek out other helping persons also. Although it is important that the doctor be aware of your wish to consult other professionals about personal or family problems, it is quite appropriate for you to take initiative in this.

In most communities, counseling and psychotherapy with individuals, families, and groups are practiced by the traditional mental health professionals: psychiatrists, clinical* psychologists and clinical or psychiatric† social workers. A growing number of psychiatric nurses, public health nurses, and clergymen with special training in pastoral counseling are also becoming effective therapists.

Of the three primary mental health professionals, only the psychiatrist is a physician, a doctor of medicine. The psychologist and professional social workers have earned master's or doctor's degrees by completing a program of formal academic study and supervised clinical experience. Fully qualified psychologists are certified (the use of the title *certified* is restricted by law to qualified persons) or licensed (a licensed practice is legally regulated). A national effort, spearheaded by professional social workers, is underway to require licensing or certification of social workers within each state. It is probable that social workers will eventually be accredited at various different levels of expertise (just as the licensed practical nurse is presently distinguished from the registered nurse). At present, the designation ACSW (Academy of Certified Social Workers) is an indication that the social worker has earned a postgraduate degree (master's or doctor's), has completed two years of supervised experience, has passed a qualifying examination, and has agreed to adhere to a code of ethics — and has thus become a member of the academy.

Unfortunately (because it creates confusion), the designation *social worker* is now used ambiguously. It may refer to an untrained (although often dedicated and compassionate) indigenous worker in an urban antipoverty program. It may be applied to a welfare department caseworker — most likely a college graduate who may (or may not) have completed courses in sociology or social welfare administration.

In a hospital, there may be a volunteer or a secretary who "does the social work," perhaps telephoning nursing homes to find vacant beds for patients being discharged. Some hospital staffs do include professional social workers who are skillful at giving assistance with practical needs: helping the family find sources of financial help, making arrangements for transportation to the hospital, helping locate homemaker services to provide care for other family members if the mother stays in the hospital with the sick child or to provide home nursing assistance when the child returns. Some hospital social workers are also skilled in personal counseling, some are not.

*The term *clinical* distinguishes practitioners engaged in person-to-person work with troubled people from those engaged in program administration, education, and research.

†The term *psychiatric* denotes special training and experience in the field of mental health.

If the staff of your child's hospital does not include fully qualified, professional social workers, you may wish to seek help at a family counseling service, a mental health center, or a child guidance clinic. Such agencies can be located through the Yellow Pages of your phone directory (under such listings as "Marital and Family Counseling," "Social Services"), through the United Fund (known also as United Way, Community Chest) office in your community, through the Visiting Nurses Association, or by writing a national headquarters (see Appendix).

Parents are often unaware that their child's hospital may include a chaplaincy service. An increasing number of hospital chaplains are trained in pastoral counseling. In some respects, the skills of such a chaplain and those of a mental health counselor are likely to be similar. A particular contribution of the chaplain-counselor, however, can be to help sick children and their families find meaning in their plight in relation to their religious beliefs. A chaplain can help explore the agonizing questions: "Is this God's punishment?" "Why was *I* chosen?" "Can I go on believing in a God who could allow this tragedy to befall us?"

Counseling is not a method of telling you what to do. Rather, it is a method of helping you explore and come to understand your feelings, attitudes, and needs — as well as those of other family members — and then helping you use your self-knowledge to make decisions and plan courses of action that suit your personality and family situation. A skilled counselor has a thorough understanding of personality development and a deep respect for individuality and the right of all persons to determine their own destinies.

Parent Groups

Parents who face a common problem and share a common need may benefit from associating with each other in various kinds of groups. The more clearly the goals of such groups can be defined, the more effective they are likely to be. The formation of a new group requires time and energy, especially if its nature is determined entirely by those parents who expect to participate. The very process of developing into a working group invariably involves a struggle for leadership, an effort to evolve goals, agree on procedures, resolve disagreements and personality conflicts, and develop a sense of unity and trust. Parents whose time and enrgy are already drained by their child's illness may prefer to seek professional leadership in developing a new group, or to join preexisting groups. Groups related to health problems are apt to follow one of two patterns.

Educational-Informational Groups

An educational group meeting offers parents a time and a place where they can seek information from a qualified person about the nature of the disorder that afflicts their child, its treatment, and the medical research directed toward finding a cure. (But such a meeting is not an appropriate substitute for individual conferences about your own child's particular needs at a particular time.)

Such groups are likely to meet on a regular basis — weekly, semimonthly or monthly — and preferably in the evening so that employed parents can participate. They are likely to be conducted by a physician, perhaps in cooperation with other health professionals, such as a nurse, dietitian, or inhalation therapist.

Such meetings may take the form of a lecture or demonstration by the professional, followed by a question period; or they may be conducted as informal discussions of information the parents request. The structure of the meeting is apt to be determined by the personality and philosophy of the physician as well as by the expressed wishes of the parents.

If the meetings are structured as lectures or demonstrations with questions, size of the group is usually not a prime consideration. However, many parents are reserved and feel shy about speaking in a large group. Discussion is usually much freer when the group is well below 20 in number.

A major hazard in such groups is that one member may ask for information that other members are not yet ready to think about. For example, at one meeting the mother of a 15-year-old boy asked the physician to confirm a new rumor that males with a certain disorder are apt to be sterile. The parents of preschool children with this disorder were shocked and grieved to be confronted with a new aspect of the illness that had been far from their thoughts. In such fashion, parents of younger children may be worried to hear of the problems of older children; parents of children with a milder form of a disorder can be frightened to learn of more severe manifestations. Unless the discussion leader is sensitive to such transmissions of anxiety and is able to remind the group that the problem afflicting one child may never become a concern to another child, the meetings can arouse more anxiety and sorrow than they assuage.

On the other hand, educational group meetings offer parents a situation in which they can absorb significant information slowly and by hearing it discussed repeatedly. Rather than suffering the embarrass-

ment of having to ask their child's physician the same question again
and again until they can assimilate the answer, they can benefit by having the same question asked by other parents. Furthermore, especially if
the discussion leader encourages parents to describe their own solutions
to everyday problems, they can profit by hearing about the variety of
helpful techniques used by others.

Finally, every parent's sense of being alone in facing awesome
problems and monumental tasks may be reduced by the presence of
others who share similar needs and concerns. Sometimes parents continue their associations informally in between meetings, often developing warm friendships and offering each other practical help. (But supportive as such friendships may be, it is usually unwise to socialize *only*
with other parents of ill children. This can lead to a preoccupation with
the illness so excessive that nothing else in life seems meaningful.)

An educational-informational group program requires medical
leadership. In a large medical center, specialists are often available and
interested in working with parents in this way. Such programs may also
be sponsored by the state department of health, the Visiting Nurses
Association or the appropriate voluntary health agency.

Experiential-Therapeutic Groups

An experiential group is one whose members meet regularly to understand and share the social and emotional experience of caring for a
child with extended illness.

Such understanding is attained by gradually uncovering and venting the feelings aroused by the child's disorder. As one parent listens to
another, he may begin to identify his own inner feelings more clearly.
With the group leader's help, he may begin to understand why painful
feelings and worrisome thoughts are aroused, and to realize that they are
prevalent among other parents. He may feel reassured that he is not unnatural or crazy, and therefore develop greater confidence in examining
and articulating his own inner experience.

In addition to the deeper awareness and acceptance of his own
feelings he may attain, and the sense of emotional affinity to others, the
parent has the opportunity to hear what approaches and techniques
other parents have found effective, or ineffective, in dealing with issues
·arising daily within the family. Therefore, his own capacity to cope may
be strengthened — and in this sense, such a group experience is truly
therapeutic.

The group requires effective leadership, usually by a mental health professional. The leader, either a psychiatrist, social worker, or psychologist, should have a deep understanding of personality development and family relationships. The leader needs to convey an acceptance of individuality, and a recognition that for different families different patterns of behavior may be appropriate and effective.

Through his own attitudes of acceptance and understanding, the leader can promote a sense of trust within the group. Members learn to feel safe in exposing their sensitive feelings without risk of criticism and harsh judgment, and thus increase their effectiveness in self-expression. Although encouraging free exchange among the parents, the leader will guide the discussion sufficiently so that it does not become fragmented into multiple conversations between two or three people, so that parents do not vent their hostilities upon each other, and so that the discussion does not remain at an unendurably sorrowful level. It is likely that the leader will arrange for separate, individual conferences with parents whose needs cannot be adequately met in the group experience.

Such a group can be effective only if size is restricted (12 to 16 members are generally considered the upper limit) and if the membership is reasonably constant. Although a well-consolidated group of a dozen members can usually absorb a few additions, it is difficult to promote a sense of group trust if the membership changes markedly with each meeting. For this same reason, clear limits must be set on the number of health professionals wishing to attend as observers.

The discussions may be extemporaneous, developing around any observation or question a parent may bring up at the start; or the group may plan with the leader to organize topical discussions around particular issues (preparing a child for hospitalization, informing relatives about the diagnosis — in fact, any one of the issues discussed in this book could become the matrix of a group discussion).

The length of each meeting should be clearly determined and rather strictly observed. An appointed beginning and end helps parents use the time effectively and avoids prolonging the meeting to the point of exhaustion. The frequency of the meeting, as well as the number planned in a given series, is likely to be recommended by the leader on the basis of prior experience, although parental preferences should be given serious consideration.

It is inevitable that some medical questions will arise during the sessions. Whether or not any of the physicians caring for the children should participate in such meetings is to a great extent dependent on the personality, skills, and interests of the physician. An experiential group is directed toward finding its own solutions from within the individual and the shared experience. Except for psychiatrists, most physicians are trained to supply answers and give direct advice, and lay people expect them to be knowledgeable and authoritative. Therefore, it may be uncomfortable for the physician and frustrating for the parents if the physician is present only as a listener and a resource person available to answer occasional questions. Furthermore, the fact that he *is* present disposes parents to focus on the physical issues rather than on the experiential ones, and even to seek consultations about their own children.

One possible compromise is for the physician to participate in one part of the meeting — perhaps a second part, after a coffee break. Questions concerning medical aspects of the disorder that have remained unanswered can then be brought to his attention. An alternative is to ask the physician to attend the first part only, and then to focus upon the social and emotional aspects of the disorder later in the meeting. Often the best solution, if it is practical, is to arrange for the two different types of meetings to be conducted separately and for parents to attend either or both.

It is not essential that the experiential meetings be conducted in a medical center. Should no adequately trained mental health professionals be available, parents may profitably seek such a group experience through a local mental health center or family counseling agency. Parents who worry that such professionals may not adequately understand the particular physical disorder might be reminded that the mental health worker can readily inform himself by consulting both the physician and the wealth of information available in professional journals.

Single-Parent Groups

Married parents seek companionship, understanding, and solace from each other. There are many marriages in which the partners fail to meet each other's needs, but if understanding and emotional intimacy are lacking, there is usually some sharing of responsibility, some practical help.

The single parent lacks even this. It can be bleak, lonely, and frightening to raise a healthy child without a marital partner — bearing full responsibility for making decisions; supplying affection and care and guidance alone; receiving the full brunt of the child's emotional storms and his strivings for independence. Much more difficult is the plight of a single parent whose child's health is seriously impaired. All the needs and tasks described in this book seem to be his to cope with alone, posing a monumental challenge that even a superparent would find overwhelming.

It is essential for the single parent to seek out every available source of help — relatives, friends, and all the professional persons mentioned throughout the book. In addition, it can be helpful to associate with others facing similar challenges.

In recent years, various associations of single people have developed. Some serve as little more than dating bureaus, exposing their members to all the physical and emotional hazards involved in sexual liaisons between virtual strangers. Some singles organizations strive to offer broad programs of social and recreational activities for unmarried persons. Some sponsor discussion groups in which problems related to being single may be examined.

The special needs of single parents are the particular concern of a few private organizations, such as Parents without Partners, Inc., Single Parents, Inc., as well as of community centers, women's centers, and family counseling agencies. Their group programs can be a source of considerable emotional support, as well as of helpful, practical information. It is important to assure yourself of the responsibility, good intent, and merit of any such group before becoming a member. Inquiries can be made within your own community of your clergyman, the United Fund, or even the chamber of commerce.

Voluntary Health Agencies

In past years, most voluntary health agencies were started by relatives and concerned friends of a person afflicted with a serious illness, such as tuberculosis, poliomyelitis, or cancer. More recently, some such organizations have started at the prompting of physicians alarmed at the dwindling away of federal funds to support medical research.

Agencies are organized at local, state, and national levels, with direct parent participation normally greatest at the local level. Excepting a few salaried workers, the manpower is voluntary, unpaid. Officers, boards of directors, and their working committees may include relatives and friends of an afflicted person, lay persons with a more general interest in health problems, professionals from medicine, social work, nursing, or the clergy. Such persons bring different perspectives and experience to the agencies, and they also bring different vested interests and feelings of urgency about particular problems. Therefore, the program emphasis may vary greatly from one agency to another. However, all such agencies engage to some degree in fund raising, research, professional education, public education, service, and social action.

Fund Raising

Since all programs of the agencies require financial support, fund raising is naturally the foundation of the agencies' work. Funds are solicited privately, either on a door-to-door basis or through the mail. (Unfortunately, as health agencies proliferate in number, they compete with each other in solicitation, and an increasing number of harassed householders have begun to refuse their appeals altogether.)

Funds are raised through subscribed events, such as dances, theatrical performances, and sports events. Appeals for funds are made through the mass media, press, radio, television. To move the reader, listener, or viewer to donate money, these appeals often dramatize to the utmost the plight of afflicted children. Parents have observed how alarming such portrayals are to the children who are exposed to them. As a consequence of parental concern, some appeals have been modified.

Funds are raised through appeals to congressmen to introduce legislation appropriating needed public funds. An outstanding example of this was the work of the Connecticut chapter of the Cooley's Anemia Blood and Research Foundation for Children in interesting a national congressman in the problems and needs of those afflicted with this disorder. The result — brought about by his work and influence in Congress — was an appropriation of federal funds.

Research

In most agencies, support of medical research is given high priority in allocation of funds. The research is not, of course, carried out by the agency itself; rather, the work of selected scientists and physicians whose programs are deemed significant by the medical advisory board (usually associated with the national board of directors) is supported through grants. Funding from The National Foundation—March of Dimes made a major contribution to the development of a vaccine preventing infantile paralysis, for example.

Professional Education

Voluntary health agencies sponsor and support professional conferences and workshops. At such meetings, physicians and related professionals have an opportunity to meet colleagues from other centers (and perhaps other lands) and learn of their research and care programs.

Some agencies support the publication of professional journals that report current advances in diagnosis and care of afflicted persons. Some agencies are able to provide financial support for the training of scientists or technicians.

Public Education

The health associations have informed the public about the causes, manifestations, and treatment of various disorders. The Epilepsy Foundation of America, for example, has helped to dispel much of the superstitious dread of this illness. The American Heart Association continues a dedicated effort to prevent rheumatic fever, a leading cause of heart disease acquired in childhood, by urging physicians and parents to have any child complaining of a sore throat tested to see if a streptococcal infection is the cause. The American Cancer Society publicizes the early signs and symptoms of that disease, in the hope that afflicted persons will seek earlier and, it is to be hoped, more effective treatment.

Some agencies publish and distribute informational pamphlets intended to help the families of children afflicted with such disorders as diabetes, leukemia, and cystic fibrosis. The pamphlets promote better understanding of the illnesses and of their complex treatments (a list of agencies is found on pages 232-233).

Service

The expenses associated with extended illness can be catastrophic. Voluntary health agencies rarely have sufficient funds to give large grants to any one family (one case might deplete the total budget of a local agency). However, some agencies are able to extend interest-free loans or to make small outright grants to help meet specific needs, such as those for home nursing, medications, or sickroom equipment. Some agencies are able to lend complex, expensive treatment apparatus. Some agencies provide a consulting and referral service to help families locate sources of financial help. For example, the executive director of the Cystic Fibrosis Association of Connecticut provided invaluable assistance in helping families gather and interpret information about their children's medical insurance coverage.

Other practical services may be offered, such as providing transportation to medical facilities and helping a family locate and transport blood donors to maintain supplies for a child with a disorder such as hemophilia or Cooley's anemia. In Chicago, an agency and a family cooperated to arrange periodic group donor sessions at which concerned relatives, friends, and acquaintances contributed blood to maintain reserves for the six hemophiliac boys in the family. Group participation gave emotional support to the donors, as well as providing them with transportation. (The family provided a banquet afterward to express their thanks.)

Screening Programs

One special form of service is the screening program, usually carried out in cooperation with public health departments, local physicians, or both. Diagnostic screening programs have included the mobile x-ray unit used to detect respiratory ailments, blood testing to detect poisonous levels of lead among young children prone to chew on inedible, and sometimes dangerous, objects, programs to detect diabetes and high blood pressure, and a variety of others.

Increasingly, screening programs are being designed to identify carriers of genetic traits that may result in inherited disorders, such as Cooley's anemia, Tay-Sachs disease, and sickle cell anemia. Such programs may be sponsored by voluntary health agencies and carried out by medical professionals. It is hoped — although evidence of the programs' effectiveness still needs to be gathered — that they will in time result in a decreased incidence of such disorders.

Genetic screening programs are now being evaluated by many thoughtful physicians, clergymen, and other professionals who are concerned about the influence of such programs on the behavior, attitudes, and emotions of the participants. It is widely agreed that in a well-run program, the public should be thoroughly informed (with ample opportunity to raise questions) about the nature of the inherited disorder, its possible dangers, and the pattern of transmission from one generation to the next. It should be informed how the birth of afflicted babies might be avoided. The public should then be offered an opportunity, hopefully free of coercion by others in their community, for individual testing to determine if the genetic trait is present.

In a well-run program, findings should be confidential. Those free of the trait should be notified for reassurance. Those bearing the trait should be informed in a personal conference with a health professional. Since emotionally charged information is usually understood and absorbed slowly, there should be follow-up conferences (either private or in a small group) in which genetic counseling can be carried out.

Social Action

A nation's most precious natural resource is its children. Certain European countries, especially those in northern and eastern Europe, have demonstrated a much higher level of national commitment to the welfare of their children than has the United States. Health programs include emphasis on early case finding, comprehensive diagnosis and planning, and organization of helping resources in or near the child's own community.

Recent studies have yielded estimates that from 10% to 12% of our children are afflicted with significant physical impairments. Their families constitute a potentially awesome source of "parent power," which can — and needs to — be used on behalf of children with extended illness.

Parents sometimes associate independently to engage in social action, perhaps working in consultation with experts in government, industry, education, and the health professions. They may also work effectively through the existing voluntary health agencies.

There are countless areas in which constructive action is needed to improve the quality of their children's lives.

Modifying the Physical Environment

Any youngster with a disorder resulting in weakness, easy fatigability, faintness, dizziness, shortness of breath, or short stature has justification for believing he lives in an uncaring world when he moves through the streets and attempts to use schools, libraries, sports arenas, theaters, and other facilities. It is well within technological and architectural capabilities to provide an environment that such a youngster (as well as the elderly and the mother pushing a baby carriage) could readily master: buildings with ramps; wide doorways and doors that open electronically; elevators with wide access and low push-buttons; low water fountains and public telephones; rest rooms with a screened-off cot for rest periods and with grab bars by the toilets; ramps at street corners; ramps leading to building entrances and connecting the stories of buildings internally; benches on long city blocks and at bus stops.

During the 1960s the Architectural Barriers Project was initiated under the sponsorship of the President's Committee on the Employment of the Handicapped and of the National Society for Crippled Children and Adults, with support from the Vocational Rehabilitation Administration. National standards were developed. In 1968, the Federal

Architectural Barriers Act was passed, requiring all federal projects and any building using federal funds to meet certain accessibility standards. Many states have developed comparable legislation. For example (largely the result of efforts of the National Federation of the Blind in Connecticut), in 1973 Connecticut passed a law barring discrimination against the blind and the physically disabled. Implementation of this law will require that the streets and public transportation be made physically accessible to handicapped persons, and it will forbid discrimination against the handicapped in either public or private employment.

Parents can scarcely redesign towns and cities. They can, however, exert influence on specific building projects. For example, when a new school or library is to be built — or an old one remodeled — a parent group could exert influence on the design by working closely with the building committee. They could, perhaps, urge the local chapter of the League of Women Voters to study and report on recent legislation (federal, state, and local) concerned with discrimination against the physically disabled, and to evaluate how such laws might effect local building codes. They could bring pressure to bear on local government to insure that existing laws are implemented.

Recreation and Travel

When theaters, concert halls, stadiums, and libraries are physically accessible to all persons, youngsters with physical impairments will be able to enjoy a wider range of those recreational opportunities available to the general public.

However, there is need for special programs as well. Few, if any, cities in the United States have followed the example of Ramat Gan (near Tel Aviv, Israel) in establishing a sports club specially equipped and programmed for those with physical impairments. There are too few camping programs available for youngsters whose medical treatment is complex and requires specialized supervision.

Some help is available for traveling with a child with impaired health. For example, Pan American was a pioneer among airlines in developing special travel programs. The American Automobile Association offers information and guidance. Furthermore, it is possible to obtain information about special facilities in particular areas by writing to the local chamber of commerce.

The literature available is likely to have such titles as, "Guide for the Handicapped." Understandably, parents of children with many health impairments — kidney, heart, lung, and blood diseases, diabetes, and epilepsy, for example — tend not to think of their children as handicapped or disabled and fail to seek such information. Although the term *handicapped* is associated with crutches or braces in many minds, in reality any child who suffers from marked weakness or faintness or shortness of breath or seizures or digestive problems does have special needs. His travels can be made more comfortable and pleasurable by advance planning.

The likelihood of obtaining appropriate medical attention can be increased also. For example, for a small fee, a child can be enrolled as a member of Medic-Alert.* He will be supplied with an emblem (to be worn on a necklace or bracelet) listing his name, file number, and an emergency phone number to which a collect call can be put through 24 hours per day. If an emergency should arise, an available physician could promptly obtain significant information about the child's disorder through such a call.

For travel abroad, an organization known as Intermedic offers a worldwide directory of English-speaking physicians and a special form on which to record significant health information.

However, these are only encouraging beginnings, and parent power could become a significant influence in achieving further progress. For example, should not all communities of interest to the tourist, as well as all state and national parks, provide information about facilities for those with health problems, and develop such facilities if they fail to exist? Should not all common carriers — buses, trains, commercial airplanes — be equipped with basic lifesaving equipment (oxygen with child-size as well as adult-size airways, for example) and with personnel trained in basic lifesaving techniques? Should not an emergency communications system be available on all major highways?

Baby-Sitters

Parents of ill children urgently need periods for recreation and replenishment and times just to be together as man and wife. However, there is often worry about whether an ill child can safely be left with a baby-sitter. One solution is for parents who live in the same community to arrange baby-sitting pools among themselves whereby they will baby-sit for each other on a reciprocal basis. Another solution is to work cooperatively with a high-school or college employment office and local physicians to arrange special training for students willing to baby-sit with ill children. The local hospital volunteer office or a community

*See Appendix.

volunteer service bureau might establish a registry of specially qualified baby-sitters. A local nursing school might establish a registry among its nursing students.

School Policies

It has been estimated that only one third of the United States are educating more than half of their physically and mentally disabled children. It is believed that one million disabled children are not in schools of any sort. Although a proportion of these are children with severe intellectual or emotional disabilities, there are also a very large number who have unimpaired psychological capacities for learning. It is likely that well under one third (perhaps far fewer) of our children with physical limitations are being adequately educated.

Seen in its overview, the dimensions of the problem appear overwhelming. However, within the individual community, using existing facilities, parents of children with extended illnesses can exert influence.

Regulations concerning homebound teaching or tutorial help, regulations concerning physical education, as well as regulations concerning the use of medications in school are all areas that may create problems and embarrassment for the school-age child with impaired health (Chapters 5 and 6). These are areas in which parent groups may be able to work effectively with school administrators and boards of education.

Medical Insurance

Some insurance companies are penny wise and pound foolish. That is, by declining to cover on an out-patient basis certain procedures covered for the hospitalized patient, the companies encourage physicians to arrange medically unnecessary admissions, subject the child to avoidable psychological stress, subject the family to disruption, and incur for themselves far larger expenses than would be required otherwise. In 1971, for example, a major insurer would not cover costs of a kidney dialysis apparatus for home use, although the expense for home treatment was estimated at around $5,000 a year (after the initial purchase of the equipment), compared to about $25,000 a year for dialysis in a hospital. Vigorous efforts to modify insurance coverage were made by the National Kidney Foundation and the National Association of Patients on Hemodialysis. Until recently, a major insurer would not cover blood transfusions on an out-patient basis, thus subjecting children with blood disorders to frequent, avoidable hospital admissions. In at least one state (Connecticut) an insurer was persuaded by a voluntary health agency (the Cooley's Anemia Blood and Research Foundation for Children) to modify its policy on a trial basis. In such fashion, parent power, allied with the influence of physicians, businessmen and politicians, can exert significant influence on private insurers.

Humanizing Hospitalization

Those concerned with the mental health of children have recognized for over 30 years that much can be done to ameliorate the emotional and social stresses to which the hospitalized child and his family are subjected. There has been progress in liberalizing visiting policies. A few hospitals have established "living-in" or "parent care" programs, in which parents are provided facilities and encouraged to remain with their hospitalized children (especially very young and critically ill children) and to participate in their care in ways that help the nursing staff and reassure the child. A few medical centers have established "day hospitals" to which children (even those with very serious disorders) come for complex medical treatment during the daytime and are permitted to return home at night (with a physician available by phone). Some hospitals have adequate, even outstanding, recreational and educational programs.

However, in the nation as a whole, facilities and programs lag far behind the recognition of need. Hospital administrators and boards of directors are giving increasing recognition to the needs and desires of the "consumer." Parent power, in alliance with medical staff, can exert significant influence.

In any such area, a group of parents interested in social action* can find a meaningful common goal. Such activity not only results in improvement of the quality of life of the child with extended illness but also provides a constructive outlet for the sense of frustration and protest — the pent-up anger and aggressive energy — that is aroused in many parents.

Financial Resources

The prolonged health problems of childhood can become a staggering drain on the financial resources of the family. Until such time as

---

*Some parents are emotionally unable to involve themselves in an action-oriented group. Such parents may find that — to replenish themselves emotionally and spiritually — they must use any free moments to engage in pursuits totally unrelated to their child's illness.

families are protected against the expenses of "catastrophic illnesses" by a national insurance plan, it may be necessary to draw on a variety of different resources. Some guidance in finding such resources should be available through your child's hospital (the admitting office, the business office, or the social service department), through the local department of welfare, through a family counseling agency, or through the appropriate voluntary health agency. The most likely sources of aid include the ones discussed below.

Medical Insurance

A surprising number of families fail to explore fully the benefits to which they are entitled under their insurance policies. Should clear information be difficult to obtain from the insuror, assistance in interpreting the policy could be sought from any of the sources mentioned above. In addition, if the family is covered by a group plan sponsored by the wage earner's business firm, clarification can be sought from that firm, perhaps through the personnel office.

State Department of Health

In most states, some funds are disbursed for the care of children with certain illnesses or disabilities through the state department of health. The programs are administered by special sections such as the division of crippled children or maternal and child health. Eligibility for the funds varies in individual states, but it is worthwhile for all families to inquire about their own eligibility. The funds, after all, are accrued from taxes to which most families have contributed.

State Vocational Rehabilitation Services

At the age of 16, youngsters become eligible for certain forms of financial aid (as well as for training and vocational counseling) from the division concerned with vocational rehabilitation. Such a division may operate with the state department of health, education, or labor.

Veterans Services

Families of veterans may be eligible for financial assistance from special funds, such as the Soldier's, Sailor's and Marine's Fund. Inquiries about available resources might be made at the information division of the local Veterans Administration.

Voluntary Health Agencies

As already has been mentioned, limited financial assistance in the form of either outright grants or interest-free loans is available through certain of the voluntary health agencies.

Private Foundations and Endowments

Concerned persons or families have bequeathed money to establish trust funds, the interest from which can be used for assistance with medical problems at the discretion of the trust officers. Information about such funds would most likely be obtained through the hospital's admitting office or social service department.

Medicaid

Under federal legislation referred to as Title XIX, Medical Assistance Program, federal funds are disbursed through the states for the medical care of children in families whose financial resources fall below a certain level. These funds are disbursed either through the state department of health or the state department of welfare (although they are not welfare monies). Inquiries about eligibility can be made at the local department of welfare office or at the hospital.

Satisfactions Outside Parenthood

Modern parents are likely to be involved in the care and rearing of their young for only one half, or less, of their adult years. As families have become smaller and adults have lived longer, many parents have become vulnerable to an emotional crisis in mid-life referred to as the "empty nest syndrome." When their children leave the nest, parents may feel adrift, lacking purpose, without a sense of worth or the fulfillment of being needed. If the marital relationship has become routine, mechanical, and unsharing, there may be little to occupy the emotional empty spaces.

Such crises may be avoided by thoughtful planning, in which it should be realized that adults, as much as children, do pass through a sequence of developmental stages. During the years of parenthood, there will be alterations in the quality and intensity of the child's needs, as well as alterations in the satisfactions parents can expect.

From his first days in school, a significant portion of a child's experience is related to places, events, and persons other than his parents. Although there are days (up to the teen years) when it is meaningful to have a parent, most likely his mother, at home to receive his first urgent communications about the joys or sadness of his day, the youngster also becomes increasingly selective about what he shares. A mother is likely to feel less rebuffed by his growing need for privacy if an increasingly significant portion of her life is involved in interests other than children. Even those mothers who prefer homemaking to any other role may find their lives enriched — and may become more effective wives and parents — by developing a special talent or by participating in community activities.

Parents of children with impaired health are likely to have especially intense needs for replenishment and satisfactions from sources other than child care. Although their affection for their child may be deep and their capacity to help him cope with his affliction may be profoundly satisfying, they must also endure the burden of chronic sorrow, struggle with pangs of remorse, and quell flashes of resentment. Furthermore, if all their satisfactions are derived from child care, even to the extreme of "desperate clinging" (Chapter 6), contemplation of loss becomes unendurable.

However, just such parents may find it especially complex to arrange meaningful outside activities. The financial drain of the illness may limit the kinds of recreational activities that can be enjoyed. If employment is sought, an employer must be found who is willing to tolerate unpredictable and perhaps frequent absenteeism when the child is acutely ill.

To some degree, all married women share the problems of finding an effective balance between meeting family needs and pursuing independent interests. An increasing number of information and counseling centers for women are developing throughout the nation, especially in communities in which there is a university. In such centers women are offered educational or career counseling. They may be guided in identifying their interests and in locating colleges that offer continuing education programs for the part-time student or the student who had interrupted her education. There is guidance in finding opportunities for satisfying volunteer work, and there may be a roster of part-time jobs with flexible requirements. There are also opportunities to meet other women sharing similar concerns. Such women's centers can be located by examining the Yellow Pages under "Associations" and "Social Services," or through inquiry at the local United Fund office or at a nearby college or university.

No outside pursuit can bring full contentment, however, if the emotional atmosphere at home is barren. Marriage in the United States is subject to its own particular strains. Because of the high degree of mobility of young families and the tendency to reject many of the values and accomplishments of the preceding generation, the family unit is likely to be isolated (physically or emotionally, or both) from kin. Husband and wife may, as a result, expect each other to serve as friend, lover, brother, sister, father, and mother; and since such expectations are unrealistic, disappointment and anger are likely to follow. Furthermore, ours is a striving, competitive society that places a high premium on visible success and acquisition of material possessions. The expectation of financial success subjects the chief wage earner to constant pressure and may demand long hours of work away from home.

Prolonged health problems in a child further strain and burden the marital relationship in a variety of ways (Chapter 2), although parents of an ill child need each other's support, solace, and encouragement above all else. It is crucial to protect the relationship, to be vigilant for signs of trouble and to seek help early, before problems erupt destructively. It is essential to arrange times that are clearly For Parents Only, whether they are for enjoying tender intimacy in the bedroom or for walking together through the forest in autumn. Before any child is born, and long after he is gone from home, there is man and woman together.

Appendix: Service Organizations

It is sometimes difficult for parents to locate sources of information and help within or near their own communities. The organizations listed below endeavor to respond appropriately to written requests for guidance.

Camping

(The following agencies either provide information or publish camp directories.)

American Camping Association, Bradford Woods, Martinsville, Indiana 46151

Association of Jewish Sponsored Camps, J.C.I.S., 130 East 59th St., New York, N.Y. 10003.

Association of Private Camps, Room 621, 55 West 42nd St., New York, N.Y. 10035

National Catholic Camping Association, 1312 Massachusetts Ave., N.W., Washington, D.C. 20005

Counseling and Psychotherapy

American Association of Marriage and Family Counselors, Inc., 225 Yale Ave., Claremont, Calif. 91711

American Association of Psychiatric Clinics for Children, 250 West 57th St., New York, N.Y. 10019

American Association of Psychiatric Services for Children, 1701 Eighteenth St., N.W., Washington, D.C. 20009

Family Service Association of America, 44 East 23rd St., New York, N.Y. 10010

National Association for Mental Health, 1800 North Kent St., Rosslyn Station, Arlington, Va. 22209

Family Planning

Association for Voluntary Sterilization, 14 West 40th St., New York, N.Y. 10018

Planned Parenthood—World Population (Information and Education Office), 810 Seventh Ave., New York, N.Y. 10019

Single Parents

Big Brothers of America, 220 Suburban Station Building, Philadelphia, Pa. 19103

Parents without Partners, Inc., 7910 Woodmont Ave., Washington, D.C. 20014

Travel

Intermedic, 777 Third Ave., New York, N.Y. 10017

Medic-Alert Foundation International, P.O. Box 1009, Turlock, Calif. 95380

Voluntary Health Agencies*

Allergy Foundation of America, 801 Second Ave., New York, N.Y. 10017

American Cancer Society, 219 East 42nd St., New York, N.Y. 10017

American Diabetes Association, 18 East 48th St., New York, N.Y. 10017

American Heart Association, 44 East 23rd St., New York, N.Y. 10010

American Lung Association, 1740 Broadway, New York, N.Y. 10019

Arthritis Foundation, 1212 Avenue of the Americas, New York, N.Y. 10036

Cooley's Anemia Blood and Research Foundation for Children, Inc., 3366 Hillside Avenue, New Hyde Park, N.Y. 11040

Epilepsy Foundation of America, Suite 406, 1828 L St., N.W., Washington, D.C. 20036

Leukemia Society of America, Inc., 211 East 43rd St., New York, N.Y. 10017

Muscular Dystrophy Associations of America, 810 Seventh Ave., New York, N.Y. 10019

National Cystic Fibrosis Research Foundation, 3379 Peachtree Rd., N.E., Atlanta, Ga. 30326

National Easter Seal Society for Crippled Children and Adults, 2023 West Ogden Ave., Chicago, Ill. 60612

*Voluntary health agencies also include regional and state chapters, which may have programs of considerable interest to parents. Local organizations concerned with sickle cell anemia and osteogenesis imperfecta have been formed. However, at this time the author is unable to determine whether national offices yet exist.

National Foundation-March of Dimes, P.O. Box 2000, 1275 Mamaroneck Ave., White Plains, N.Y. 10602

National Hemophilia Foundation, 25 West 39th St., New York, N.Y. 10018

National Kidney Foundation, 116 East 27th St., New York, N.Y. 10016

National Society for the Prevention of Blindness, 79 Madison Ave., New York, N.Y. 10016

United Cerebral Palsy Associations, 66 East 34th St., New York, N.Y. 10016

Women's Services

Directory entitled *Continuing Education and Related Services for Women,* U.S. Government Labor Department Pamphlet #10, Superintendent of Documents, Government Printing Office, Washington, D.C. 20402

Index

Abortion, 178-179
    after amniocentesis, 182
    laws concerning, 178-179
Accomplishment, 101-110
    creative, 107-108
    physical, 106-107
    scholastic, 103-106
Adolescence, 135-171
    bodily disorders in, 137-140
    challenges of, 136-144
    hospitalization in. *See* Hospitalization, in adolescence
    impaired health in, 135-171
        imparting information in, 147-149
        parents' feelings in, 146-147
        parents' support in, 144-161
    independence in, 140-142
    kinship in, 149-153
    preparation for problems in, 144-146
    recreational needs in, 150-151
Adolescent division, in hospital, 164-166
Adoption, 182-183
Amniocentesis, 180
Anger, of parents, 9-13
    toward church, 10-11
    discharge of, 11-12
    toward doctors and nurses, 10
    toward family, 9
Anxiety, of parents, 13-19
    effects of, 13-16
    mastery of, 16-18
Apprehension, 13-19. *See also* Anxiety
Architectural Barriers Act, 222-223
Artificial insemination, 183-184
Assertiveness, of infant, 47-50
Autosomes, 206
Avoidance, school, 104-106

Baby, additional. *See* Family planning
Baby-sitters
    for ill child, 224-225
    for infant, 38
Behavioral mastery, 102-103
Blame for illness, self
    in adolescents, 147-148
    in children, 115-116
    in grandparents, 33

by parents, 21-22, 191-192
    in siblings, 27-28
Bodily discharge, 11-12, 101. *See also* Movement
Body image
    of adolescent, 136
    in early childhood, 65-67
    illness and, 66-67
    play and, 76
Body maturation, 136-140. *See also* Sexual maturation
Brothers. *See* Siblings of ill child

Camps, 100, 126, 150
Career choice. *See* Occupational choice
Carriers, genetic, 208
Chaplain-counselor, 213. *See also* Clergy
Childhood. *See* Early childhood; Midchildhood
Chores, in mid-childhood, 108-110
Chromosomes, 205
Clergy, 34, 56, 90, 101, 127, 131, 150, 166-167
Clothing, for impaired adolescent, 152
Communication
    in early childhood, 72-75
    impaired, during illness, 24-25
    between physician and parents, 186-191
        medical terms and, 188-189
        nonverbal cues in, 190
Concealment versus disclosure, of physical disorder, 96-98, 125-126, 151
Conformity, in mid-childhood, 94-95
Consent to research
    by child, 200-201
    by parent, 199-200
Contraception, 175-176
Coping style, differences in, 22-23
Counseling
    agencies for, 231
    genetic, 209-211
    personal, 211-213

Daydreaming. *See also* Fantasy
  prolonged, adolescent, 139
  solace in childhood, 107
Death
  aftermath of, 203-205
  concepts of
    in adolescence, 163
    in early childhood, 68-69
    in mid-childhood, 118, 129
  conference with doctor concerning,
    202-203
  discussion of, 117-120
Denial
  of diagnosis, by parent, 1, 187-188
  of disorder
    in adolescence, 155-156
    in mid-childhood, 125-126
Development, illness and, 46
Diagnosis, response to, 1-19, 186-191
Dietary regulation
  in adolescence, 154-155
  in infancy, 39-42
Dietitian, 40, 58, 155, 193
Difference, in mid-childhood, 93-101
Discipline, 51, 102. *See also* Impulse
    control
Disclosure of disorder, to friends,
    96-98, 125-126, 151
Doctor. *See* Physician
Driver's license, 157-158

Early childhood, 54-91
  family relations in, 59-64
  hospitalization in. *See* Hospital-
    ization, in early childhood
  independence in, 59-61
  language skills in, 72-75
  protection during, 80-81
  social relationships in, 78-82
  thoughts and concepts in, 64-72
Education. *See also* School
  of handicapped, 225
  homebound, 159
  public, 220
Educational-informational groups,
    214-215
Emotional stress
  physiological effects of, 15
  psychological effects of, 13-14
  reactions to. *See* Hospitalization
Empty nest syndrome, 228

Environmental modifications, for
    handicapped, 222-223
Experiential-therapeutic groups,
    215-217
Explanation of illness
  in early childhood, 70-71, 81
  information in, 113-117
  means of, 111-113
  in mid-childhood, 110-120
  need for, 110
  to siblings, 25-26
Extension of life, 168

Family planning, 173-184. *See also*
    Genetic counseling; Inherited
    illness
  agencies for, 231-232
  extended illness of child and,
    173
  parents' needs and, 173-174
  prenatal diagnosis and, 180-181
  prevention of pregnancy in, 175-178
  termination of pregnancy in. *See*
    Abortion
Family relationships
  in adolescence, 140-141, 169-171
  after artificial insemination, 184
  after death of child, 204-209
  in early childhood, 59-64
    illness and, 61-64
  irritability in, 9
  safeguarding of, 21-35
Fantasy. *See also* Early childhood,
    thoughts and concepts in
  concerning hospitalization, 82-83
  creativity and, 72
  in "family triangle," 59-61
  language development and, 72-73
Father
  consultation by, with physician,
    190-191
  isolation of, during illness, 23
Feeding, of infant, 39-42
  encouragement of, 39-41
  restriction of, 41-42
Feelings, release of, 101, 112-113
  through creativity, 72, 101, 108, 167
  before hospitalization, 88
  during hospitalization, 90, 132
  through play, 77-78, 88, 91, 101.
    See also Bodily discharge

through verbal expression, 11, 72, 74, 101, 150
Fertility, 145
Fetoscopy, 181
Financial resources, 226-228
Food sharing, adolescent, 152
Fund raising, by voluntary health agencies, 219

Genes, 205
  dominant, 206
  heterozygous, 206
  homozygous, 206
  recessive, 206, 207-208
Genetic counseling, 209-211
Genetic screening, 221
Goal determination, in adolescence, 158-161
Grandparents of ill child, 32-35
  contributions of, 34
  responses of, 32-33
Grief
  care of baby and, 37-38
  in child, 101
  in parents, 3-4
  in siblings, 31-32
Group meetings
  of hospitalized adolescents, 165-166
  of parents. *See* Parent groups
Guilt, 4-8. *See also* Blame for illness
  coming to terms with, 8
  negative feelings and, 6-8, 52, 55, 58, 64, 170
  responsibility for illness and, 5-6, 90, 128

Health organizations, voluntary. *See* Voluntary health organizations
Home treatment
  of infant, 47-50
  procedures in, 194-195
Hope, 195-196
  in adolescence, 148
  in childhood, 117, 132-133
  research and, 197-198
Hospitalization
  in adolescence, 161-168
    activity programs in, 167
    fears in, 163
    helpful measures in, 164-168

response to, 163-164
    staff relationships in, 166-167
    stress in, 161-163
    visits in, 167-168
  in early childhood, 82-91
    preparation for, 86-89
    response to, 84-86
    stress in, 82-84
    visits in, 89-90
  humanization of, 226
  of infant, 53-58
    aftermath of, 58
    communication with staff in, 56-58
    responses to, 54-57
    separation in, 53-54
    visits in, 55-56
  in mid-childhood, 127-133
    preparation for, 130-131
    reactions to, 129-130
    sources of help in, 131-132
    stress in, 127-129
    sustaining hope in, 132-133
Household responsibility, in mid-childhood, 108-110

Identification, with others with disorder, 100-101
Identity, loss of, in hospital, 161
Illness
  differences caused by, 96-97
  explanation of. *See* Explanation of illness
  inherited. *See* Inherited illness
  responsibility for, 5-6, 191-192. *See also* Blame for illness, self
  theories, of
    in adolescence, 147-148
    in early childhood, 67-68
    in mid-childhood, 113-115
Impulse control, in infancy, 50-53.
    See also Assertiveness
  development of, 50-52
  in mid-childhood, 102-103
  parents and, 52-53
  playmates and, 79
  See also Discipline
Independence. *See also* Assertiveness
  in adolescence, 140-142, 153-154
  encouragement of, 157-158
  bodily disorders and, 141-142
  in early childhood, 59-61

Independence — *Continued*
  in mid-childhood, 93-94, 126
  illness and, 61-64
Infant, ill, 37-58
  assertiveness of, 47-50
  assistance in care of, 38
  communication with, 45-46
  feeding of. *See* Feeding, of infant
  home treatment of, 47-50
  hospitalization of. *See* Hospitalization, of infant
  impulse control in, 50-53
  movement and activity by, 42-46
  needs of, 37-39
Information
  flow of, from physician, 186-191
    factors interfering with, 187-189
  value of, 187
Informed consent, to research, 199-200
Inhalation therapist, 48, 58, 88, 125
Inherited illness, 21, 175, 205-209
  dominant genes in, 206-207
  recessive genes in, 207-208
  sex-linked, 209
Insurance, medical. *See* Medical insurance
Irritability, family, 9

Jobs, for teenagers, 157

Kinship, for impaired adolescent, 149-153

Language development, 72-75
Learning problems, 105
Life-extending procedures, 168
Life-style, illness and, 23-24

Marriage
  adolescent children and, 169-171
  safeguarding of, during illness, 21-25, 169-171
Maturation, sexual. *See* Sexual maturation
Medicaid, 228
Medical insurance, 227
  for out-patients, 225-226
Medical terms, comprehension of, 188-189
Medical treatment. *See* Hospitalization; Treatment

Mid-childhood, 93-133
  accomplishment in, 101-110
  explaining illness in. *See* Explanation of illness
  medical management in, 120-127
  understanding of, 120-122
Movement, of infant, 43-46. *See also* Bodily discharge
  importance of, 43-44
  passive, 45
  program development for, 44-46

Negative feelings, guilt and, 6-8
Nurse
  hospital, 56-58, 88-91, 131, 150, 166-167
  psychiatric, 212
  public health, 48, 50, 58, 125, 212
  school, 98, 100

Occupational choice, 142-144, 158-161
  guidance in, 159-161
  impaired health and, 143, 158-161
Occupational therapist, 45
Odds
  in inherited illness, 207-208
  for survival, 196
Overprotection, 81-82
  of adolescent, 156-157

Parent groups, 213-218
  educational-informational, 214-215
  experiential-therapeutic, 215-217
  single-, 217-218, 232
Peer groups. *See also* Parent groups
  in adolescence, 149-153
  in mid-childhood, 93-95
Physician
  adolescent patient and, 149, 154, 166-167
  development of partnership with, 185-186
  emotional conflicts with, by parents, 189-190
  information from, 44, 48, 50, 58, 70, 80, 87-88, 90, 98, 106, 125, 131 149-150, 186-191
  with primary responsibility, 185-186
Physiotherapist, 45, 48, 58, 125, 193
Play
  in early childhood, 75-78

during hospitalization, 91
illness and, 50, 77-78
in infancy, 46, 50
  encouragement of, 46
learning and, 76
self-expression and, 76-77
social aspects of, 78-79
Play therapist, 38, 56, 70, 89, 91
Pregnancy
by artificial insemination, 183-184
assessing outcome of, 180-181
interruption of. *See* Abortion
prevention of, 175-178
  by contraception, 175-176
  by sterilization, 176-178
Premarital sex, 137
Prenatal diagnosis, 180-181
Preparation. *See* Hospitalization
Privacy
loss of, in hospital, 161-162
in medical conference, 189
Psychologist, 38, 46, 71
Psychiatrist, 18, 71, 149
Psychotherapy, 209-211
agencies for, 231
Puberty. *See* Sexual maturation
Public education, 220

Rebellion, adolescent, 140-141
Recovery, fear of, 163
Recreation, for handicapped, 223
Recurrence of disorder. *See* Inherited
  illness
Rehabilitation counselor, 45, 160
Research, medical, 196-202
child's consent for, 200-201
informed consent for, 199-200
participation in, 198-200
preparation for, 201-202
Responsibility for illness, 5-6, 191-192.
  See also Blame for illness, self
Rivalry, in early childhood, 59-61

Satisfaction outside parenthood,
  228-230
School
avoidance of, 104-106
coping with difference at, 98-100
Screening programs, genetic, 221
Self-care, 59, 63
in adolescence, 153

during hospitalization, 91
Self-expression, play and, 76-77
Separation
in early childhood, 83
during infancy, 53-54
significance of, 53-54
Service organizations, 231-233
Sex-linked inherited illness, 209
Sexual maturation, 136-140
delayed, informing child of, 148
effect of, on health problems,
  144-145
extended illness and, 138
medical treatment and, 124-125
Siblings of ill child, 25-32. *See also*
  Family planning
after death of child, 204-205
grief reactions of, 31-32
guilt feelings of, 27-28
informing of, 25-27
reassurance of, 28-29
resentments of, 25-31
Single-parent groups, 217-218, 232
Sisters. *See* Siblings of ill child
Social action, for handicapped,
  222-226
Social relationships
in adolescence, 149-153
in early childhood, 78-82
illness and, 78-82
in mid-childhood, 93-95
Social worker, 56-57, 71, 89, 90-91,
  101, 104, 127, 131, 150, 166-167
  212-213
Speech development, 72-75
Sperm bank, 177
Sports, in mid-childhood, 106-107
State health and vocational services,
  227
Sterility, informing child of, 148-149
Sterilization, 176-178
of female, 176-177
legality of, 177
of male, 176
reversal of, 177

Teacher
homebound, 99
hospital, 131
nursery school, 38, 71, 91
school, 98-99, 101, 104, 127, 150

Teenagers. *See* Adolescence
Telephone, value of
  during hospitalization, 90, 168,
  to impaired adolescent, 151
Television, for ill children, 78
Tenderness, in early childhood, 59-61
Thought
  in adolescence, 144, 147
  in mid-childhood, 113-114
  in young children, 64-65
Trait, genetic, 206
Travel programs, for handicapped,
    223-224, 232
Treatment
  acceptance of, factors in, 193-195
  in home. *See* Home treatment
  in mid-childhood
    abandonment of, 126-127
    independence in, 122-124
    special problems in, 124-127

  understanding in, 120-122
  noncompliance in, 195
  reasons for, 192-193

Ultrasound prenatal diagnosis, 180

Veterans service, 227-228
Visiting, hospital
  of adolescents, 167-168
  of infants, 55-56
  of young children, 89-90
Vocational guidance, 159-161
Voluntary health organizations, 50,
    150, 218-221, 228, 232-233
  educational services of, 219-220
  fund raising by, 219
  practical services of, 220-221
  screening programs of, 221

Women's services, 232